Christian Mayer

Functional effects of flecainide and amiodarone

Christian Mayer

Functional effects of flecainide and amiodarone

Antiarrhythmic drugs and their effects on heart muscle activity

ScienciaScripts

Imprint
Any brand names and product names mentioned in this book are subject to trademark, brand or patent protection and are trademarks or registered trademarks of their respective holders. The use of brand names, product names, common names, trade names, product descriptions etc. even without a particular marking in this work is in no way to be construed to mean that such names may be regarded as unrestricted in respect of trademark and brand protection legislation and could thus be used by anyone.

Cover image: www.ingimage.com

This book is a translation from the original published under ISBN 978-620-2-21866-5.

Publisher:
Sciencia Scripts
is a trademark of
Dodo Books Indian Ocean Ltd. and OmniScriptum S.R.L publishing group

120 High Road, East Finchley, London, N2 9ED, United Kingdom
Str. Armeneasca 28/1, office 1, Chisinau MD-2012, Republic of Moldova, Europe
Managing Directors: Ieva Konstantinova, Victoria Ursu
info@omniscriptum.com

Printed at: see last page
ISBN: 978-620-8-83114-1

Acknowledgements

In order to write this thesis, it was necessary to familiarise myself with new working methods and to learn them. It also gave me a very interesting insight into basic research. During my work, I had to rely on various people working in the field, who provided me with advice and support and gave me the necessary basics and, last but not least, the joy and motivation to work. I would therefore like to thank my first supervisor Ass.Prof. Priv.-Doz. Dr Egbert Bisping for his professional guidance throughout the entire period of my work and for bringing me closer to the interpretation of the results. I would also like to thank my second supervisor Natasa Djalinac, MSc, with whom I spent many, often amusing, hours together in the laboratory and who taught me both working techniques and problem-solving skills, especially at the beginning. I would also like to thank Dr Ewald Kolesnik, who was able to inspire me to choose a topic in basic research and was always willing to listen to my questions. I would also like to thank the entire cardiac surgery department for the smooth cooperation, without which it would not have been possible to write this thesis.

Last but not least, I would also like to thank my friends and family, who have been so understanding and supportive, not only during the labour-intensive period of writing this thesis, but also throughout my studies. Special thanks also to Clemens Oppeck, whom I got to know through this degree programme, for a wonderful friendship.

Summary

Flecainide and amiodarone are both important drugs in the treatment of arrhythmias, especially the frequently occurring atrial fibrillation. Flecainide is in principle a drug of first choice for this indication, as it has very good conversion and low relapse rates in long-term therapy. However, it is contraindicated in people with structural heart disease and severely reduced left ventricular function, which is often the case in this patient population. Amiodarone has its place here, as it has no negative influence on cardiac activity. Nevertheless, the direct systolic and diastolic effects of these two drugs are still insufficiently known, which is why they were investigated in this study using human atrial myocardium.

The present study showed that flecainide mediates a negative inotropic effect in the human atrial myocardium and also significantly impairs the force-frequency relationship (FFR), an important physiological adaptation mechanism. In addition, an induced relaxation disorder could also be demonstrated. Inhibition of SERCA activity could be responsible as a possible mechanism for this. Amiodarone, on the other hand, appears to have a negative inotropic effect, primarily due to its solvent. Its own substance-specific effects are only present in the medium concentration range. Even at submaximal concentrations, however, amiodarone does not cause a deterioration in CFB. Similarly, diastolic function was not influenced by amiodarone.

The results of this study are thus well compatible with clinical observations and are consistent with the increased mortality under flecainide therapy in heart failure after myocardial infarction. They also confirm the good tolerability of amiodarone in heart failure. They also suggest that diastolic function should be monitored regularly during flecainide therapy and that good heart rate control should be aimed for. For amiodarone, on the other hand, the use of a solvent with less cardiodepressive properties would prove advantageous.

Table of contents

CHAPTER 1

Introduction

1.1 Physiology of heart muscle contraction

In order to properly understand and interpret the experiments carried out for this thesis and their results, it is important to know the underlying physiological processes of cardiac muscle contraction. On the one hand, this involves an electrophysiological process, where and how the action potential is generated in the cells, and on the other hand the electromechanical coupling, how this electrochemical activity is converted into mechanical activity.

1.1.1 The action potential

The heart generates the impulses required for contraction by means of autonomous stimulus generation. It is able to do this via special cardiomyocytes, which form the heart's excitation generation and conduction system. The primary pacemaker in this system is the sinus node located at the junction of the right superior vena cava. The excitation is then transmitted from this to the AV node, His bundle, Tawara bundle and Purkinje fibres - and from these the excitation is finally transmitted to the working myocardium. This leads to a coordinated depolarisation of the cardiomyocytes, which are connected to each other by gap junctions[8].

This autonomous stimulus generation in the pacemaker cells is made possible by special hyperpolarisation-activated cyclic nucleotide-gated cation channels (HCN channels), which are only expressed in these cells and through which Na^{+} and K^{+} ions enter the cells. In contrast, voltage-dependent sodium channels (Na^{+} channels) are expressed in the working myocardium. These are responsible for the rapid upstroke of the action potential, which is measurable in cells of the working myocardium in comparison to the pacemaker cells[(9)'11].

The inflowing ions lead to an increase in the open probability of voltage-gated calcium channels (vgCaCh) of the L-type (LTCC) and Ga^{2+} ions flow into the myocytes. The influx of calcium causes the cardiac ryanodine receptor (RyR2), which is located in the membrane of the sarcoplasmic reticulum (SR), to open. The SR serves the myocytes as an intracellular Ca^{2+}store[10]. The influx of cations subsequently leads to membrane depolarisation, which is now positively charged. In addition, the Ca^{2+} ions are available for electromechanical coupling and contraction, as they play an essential role there[11'13].

The inflowing ions subsequently lead to the activation of voltage-dependent potassium channels (K^{+} channels), which now transport K^{+} out of the cell, which finally terminates the action potential. The sodium in the cell is transported back into the extracellular space via the sodium-potassium ATPase (Na /K^{++} -ATPase). It also ensures that the K^{+} that has left the cell re-enters it. The $Ca^{2+}$is removed from the cytoplasm in two different ways, firstly via the sodium-calcium exchanger (NCX), which pumps Ca^{2+}out of the cell in exchange for sodium[9]and secondly via the sarcoplasmic reticulum Ca^{2+}ATPase (SERCA), which transports the Ca^{2+}back into the SR[(12)'13]. This has also been identified as the dominant mechanism in healthy hearts. The relationship also appears to shift even further in favour of SERCA at higher frequencies, and disruption of this mechanism appears to be one of the key causes of the compromised force-frequency relationship in heart failure[(14)'15]. SERCA activity is influenced by the regulatory protein phospholamban (PLB). Unphosphorylated, it acts as an inhibitor of SERCA. However, when it is phosphorylated via a cAMP-dependent (activated by ß-receptors) or a Ca^{2+}-calmodulin-dependent signalling pathway, it loses its inhibitory function[72].

1.1.2 Electromechanical coupling

Electromechanical coupling refers to the mediation of the electrical process of depolarisation in the mechanical process of contraction. As already mentioned, Ca^{2+}plays a major role in this process. The contractile unit of a (heart) muscle consists of the proteins actin, myosin, tropomyosin and troponin. Muscle contraction takes place through a conformational change in the myosin molecule, which interacts with the actin filament, causing the cell to shorten. In the resting state, however, the binding site of the actin is blocked by the troponin-tropomyosin complex. This is where the Ca^{2+}previously released into the cytosol comes into play. By docking to troponin C, it dissolves and the binding site becomes free.

The $Ca^{2+}$is then eliminated from the cytosol again by the mechanisms described in the previous chapter 1.1.1 and the heart muscle can (temporarily) relax again[(16)-17]. These processes described in Chapter 1.1.1 and 1.1.2 are illustrated in Figure 1.

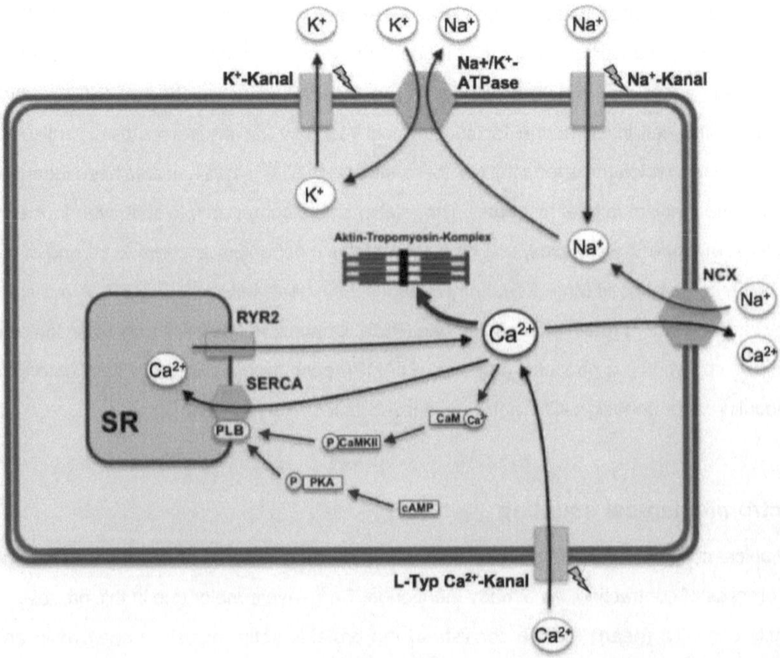

Figure 1: Schematic representation of the ionic currents and electromechanical coupling of a cardiomyocyte. Voltage-dependent Na^+ -, K^+ -, and Ca^{2+}channels are opened as part of the action potential and lead to ion influx or efflux. In addition, $Ca^{2+}$is released from the SR into the cytosol. This can now dock to the actin-tropomysion complex, allowing myosin to bind to actin and the entire muscle cell to contract. The Na /K^{++} - ATPase then restores the original ion ratios by exchanging intracellular Na^+ with extracellular IC. The SERCA and the NCX transport Ca^{2+}out of the cytosol again. SERCA can be regulated, for example, via calmodulin (CaM) and protein kinase A (PKA), which is activated via cAMP. These phosphorylate PLB, which then loses its inhibitory function on SERCA.

1.2 Inotropy and regulatory mechanisms

The process of the heart increasing or adapting its beating force is called inotropy. The inotropy of the heart can be increased or decreased by various stimuli. These can be of a nervous, hormonal or pharmacological nature. In addition, there are specific mechanisms of the heart muscle tissue such as the Frank-Starling mechanism and the force-frequency relationship, which will be discussed in more detail here[66].

1.2.1 The force-frequency relationship

One way for the heart to increase its inotropy is by changing its heart rate. This relationship is known as the force-frequency relationship of the heart. In a healthy myocardium, the myocardial contraction force increases with increasing heart rate, which is an important regulatory mechanism for myocardial and circulatory function. This effect also counteracts another negative inotropic effect. At higher heart rates, the end-diastolic filling volume decreases, as the time the heart has to refill with blood is reduced. The positive force-frequency relationship compensates or even overcompensates for this[26].

At the subcellular level, the increased loading of the SR with Ca^{2+}plays a decisive role in this mechanism. It has been shown that SERCA activity, which pumps calcium back into the SR, also increases with higher stimulation frequencies. The negative CFB in insufficient hearts and the proven ratio of Ca^{2+}elimination of SERCA and NCX in favour of NCX suggest the relevance of increasing SERCA activity for a positive CFB[(14) -27].

It has also been shown that an increase in stimulation frequency also increases the open probability of voltage-gated calcium channels. This allows additional $Ca^{2+}$to enter the cell, which is then available again for contractile function. This effect is also modified by catecholamines or inhibited by β- and calcium channel blockers. Furthermore, this mechanism appears to be impaired in the insufficient heart[28].

1.2.2 The Frank-Starling mechanism

Another possibility for increasing inotropy is the Frank-Starling mechanism, which is triggered by an increased preload or afterload (increased pre-stretching of the heart muscle cells). This mechanism enables the heart to adapt the ejection fraction to the venous return flow so that approximately the same amount of blood is pumped out of the heart as is pumped in[29].

This mechanism is mediated by an increase in the Ca^{2+}sensitivity of the myofilaments triggered by stretching of the muscle cells. The giant protein titin, which actually gives the muscle elasticity and stability, appears to play a key role in this process. However, it also appears to be able to regulate the conformation and proximity of actin and myosin, as well as the formation of cross-bridge connections of the myosin filament and the Ca^{2+}-sensitive areas of the actin filament[29].

1.3 Antiarrhythmic pharmacotherapy

The two substances investigated in this study are each antiarrhythmic drugs with different mechanisms of action, which is why this substance class and its electrophysiological effects will be briefly discussed here. According to Vaughan and Williams, antiarrhythmic drugs are categorised into classes I, II, III and IV according to their different points of action. They modify different phases of the cardiac action potential and can therefore suppress arrhythmias[40]. Class I antiarrhythmics, which are further divided into the subclasses Ia, Ib and Ic according to their kinetics and their precise electrophysiological effects, inhibit the fast voltage-dependent Na^+ channel (INS) and therefore modify the depolarisation phase (phase 0). Class II are ß-blockers, which have a negative chronotropic and dromotropic effect due to their anti-adrenergic action, also prolong the effective refractory period and thus intervene in the resting phase (phase 4). Class III antiarrhythmic drugs block various outwardly directed K^+ channels (I_K) and thus prolong the repolarisation phase (phase 3) and the effective refractory period. Last but not least, class IV antiarrhythmic drugs block the L-type voltage-gated Ca^{2+}channels ($I_{(Ca)(L)}$), thereby slowing AV conduction and modifying the plateau phase (phase 2) of the action potential[(8) '40]. Figure 2 illustrates the various points of action of an antiarrhythmic drug on the basis of an action potential.

However, it should be noted that the different substances are relatively inhomogeneous even within a class, as antiarrhythmic drugs usually act on more than one type or ion channel class. An attempt to make this more transparent was made with the "Sicilian Gambit", in which the individual substances are listed in a table and the respective effects and points of action are shown for each one[67].

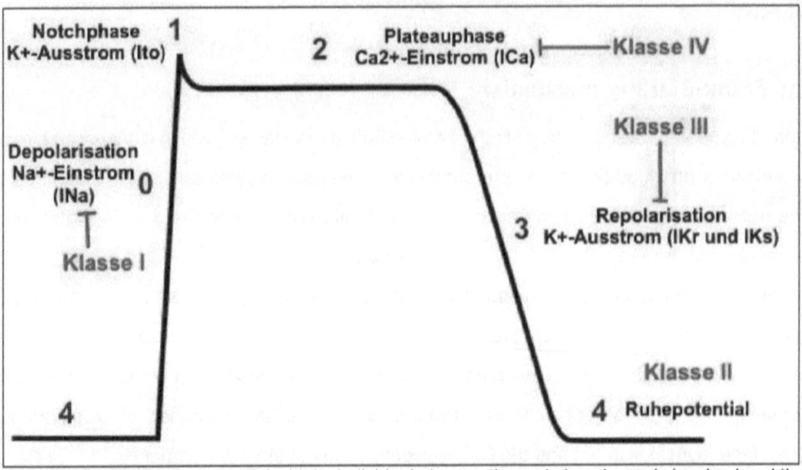

Figure 2: Cardiac action potential with its individual phases, the main ion channels involved and the points of action of antiarrhythmic drugs.

1.3.1 The class Ic antiarrhythmic agent flecainide

Flecainide, as a class Ic antiarrhythmic agent, mediates its antiarrhythmic effect via a potent selective blockade of the inwardly rectifying fast voltage-dependent Na^+ channels. This results in a flatter and longer phase 0 of the action potential. This effect only affects the working myocardium, as the pacemaker cells have HCN channels instead of Na^+ channels. Another mechanism of action is the blockade of the outwardly directed K^+ channels, especially the fast iKr channel, which are responsible for the termination of the action potential and therefore prolong it. These electrophysiological processes manifest themselves in the surface ECG via PQ, QRS and QT time prolongations[18]. An effect on the ryanodine receptor RyR2 has also been discussed[19], due to the efficacy of flecainide in catecholaminergic polymorphic ventricular tachycardia (CPVT), but this has not been confirmed[20].

Flecainide and other class Ic antiarrhythmic drugs were discredited by the CAST trial (Clinical Arrhythmia Suppression Trial), among others, as significantly more people died in the treatment group, mostly due to sudden cardiac death, than in the plecebo group[22]. Since then, despite good efficacy, restrictions have been placed on people with structural or ischaemic heart disease[18].

Nevertheless, fleceinide, along with propefenone, is in principle a first-line drug for the medical restoration of sinus rhythm in atrial fibrillation in the absence of structural heart disease[(18) '21]. Here it performed better than propefenone (72%) and amioderone (64%) with conversion rates of 90% within a 12-hour observation period[24]. In the absence of structural or ischaemic cardiac remodelling, it is suitable for the long-term therapy of persistent atrial fibrillation[21]and, with a reperfusion rate of 38%, is also better than propefenone (61%) and amioderone (47%)[23]. It is very well suited to the therapy of a "pill in the pocket", where the patient takes a larger oral dose when he/she notices the cardiac arrhythmia. This method has so far proved to be only minimally worse than the Krenkenheus Kerdioversion and successes have been achieved in 94% of arrhythmias and 84% of patients. This effectively reduced hospitelisations and saved resources[(18) '21].

Other indications for which flecainide is used are supraventricular tachycardias (SVTs) such as AV nodal reentry tachycardia (AVNRT) and atrioventricular reentry tachycardia (AVRT), for which, however, other often more favourable treatment methods also exist. The indications for ventricular tachycardia (VT) are very limited, not least because of the often underlying structural heart disease. However, one example would be right ventricular outflow tract tachycardia[18]. Rare indications for which flecainide is used as first line therapy are the aforementioned CPVT[19]and foetal supraventricular tachycardia[25].

When using flecainide, it is important to be aware of its side effects. In rare cases, its proarrhythmogenic effect can also trigger ventricular tachycardia (VTs) in healthy hearts (< 3% in cardioversions). More frequently, however, it can favour the development of atrial flutter with rapid 1:1 conduction (3.5-5%). This can be counteracted by using substances that inhibit AV conduction, such as beta-blockers, verapamil or diltiazem. Like many other antiarrhythmic drugs, flecainide also has a negative inotropic effect, which makes it unattractive and dangerous in people with heart failure or reduced ejection fraction (EF)[18].

Knowing the good efficacy and knowing the possible side effects, one should pay attention to certain things when using this drug. These include closely monitoring patients, especially at the start of therapy, and carrying out regular ECG checks during the first few days until the appropriate therapeutic dose is reached to detect abnormalities and rule out an increase in QRS duration of more than 25%. Furthermore, ischaemic and structural heart disease, impaired left ventricular EF, high-grade AV block, other conduction disturbances and other contraindications should be excluded[(18) '23].

1.3.2 The class III antiarrhythmic drug amiodarone

According to the Vaughan Williams classification, amiodarone is categorised as a class III antiarrhythmic drug and acts primarily by inhibiting the K^+ channels. This causes a prolongation of phase 3 of the action potential and an extension of the effective refractory period. In the ECG, this sometimes manifests itself in a prolongation of the QT time. However, the mechanism of action of amiodarone is complex and is still not understood down to the last detail. As a "dirty drug", in addition to K^+ channel blockade, it also has antiarrhythmic class I, II and IV properties. It can therefore also have a bradycardicising (class II), P-R time prolonging (class IV) or QRS complex widening (class I) effect[48 50].

It is used because of its good efficacy in both ventricular and supraventricular (tachy) arrhythmias. In addition, especially in comparison with other antiarrhythmic drugs, it has a very low proarrhythmogenic potency and a less pronounced or almost non-existent negative inotropic effect[48]. There are even publications in which a positive effect on left ventricular pump function (LVEF) has been shown[52], which is why amiodarone is often the only possible option, especially in people with heart failure or compromised ventricular function.

However, what complicates the use of amiodarone is its very specific pharmacokinetics. It is highly lipophilic and accumulates very strongly in the tissue. With prolonged therapy, the half-life after discontinuation is between 60 and 142 days. In addition, absorption is incomplete and varies from individual to individual (bioavailability: 30-70%). In addition, it must first be topped up at the start of therapy until it reaches its optimum efficacy (loading)[48]. The strong lipophilicity is also the reason why injection solutions must also contain a solubiliser consisting of the polysorbate "Tween 80" and benzyl alcohol.

A further problem with the use of amiodarone is its numerous extracardiac side effects and interactions with other medications, which often makes amiodarone a second choice therapeutic agent for patients without heart failure. The side effects very frequently include micro-deposits on the cornea (90%) and disorders of thyroid metabolism due to the high iodine content of amiodarone. The rare but usually very serious side effects on the lungs (pulmonary fibrosis 2%) should also be emphasised. Side effects can also occur in the skin, liver and CNS. In principle, the likelihood and severity of side effects increase with the dose and duration of therapy. For this reason, amiodarone therapy should always be closely monitored and any organs that may be affected should be checked regularly[49].

Nevertheless, amiodarone is an essential drug in the treatment of many arrhythmias, especially in individuals with compromised LVEF. It is currently used for rhythm control and off-label for rate control in atrial fibrillation when other antiarrhythmic drugs are contraindicated[21]. In principle, it is not the drug of first choice for cardioversion, but it can be given additionally before and after cardioversion and catheter ablation to maximise therapeutic success. In the prevention of ventricular arrhythmias, it is inferior to implantable cardioverter defibrillators (ICDs), but is often an important alternative if this is not possible or desirable. In emergency medicine, it is important in patients with severe cardiovascular impairment and has its own position in the resuscitation algorithm[48 51].

1.4 Questions and aims of the work

- What are the inotropic and lusitropic effects of the antiarrhythmic drugs flecainide and amiodarone in isolated human atrial myocardium?
- What are the effects on diastolic function?
- How is the force-frequency relationship influenced by these antiarrhythmic drugs?
- What is the relationship between specific substance effects and non-specific solvent effects?
- What mechanisms explain the functional effects of the two antiarrhythmic drugs studied?

CHAPTER 2

Material and methods

All experiments performed for this thesis were carried out with isolated myocardial trabeculae from the human right heart ear. In total, tissue from 29 hearts was obtained for this work, and measurements were carried out on 61 trabeculae.

2.1 Buffer and nutrient solutions

2.1.1 Tyrode solution

In order to create the best possible conditions for the trabeculae in the organ bath of the test facility, it was filled with a so-called Tyrode solution (modified Krebs-Henseleit buffer). In order to come as close as possible to physiological conditions, the solution is gassed with carbogen (95% O_2, 5% CO2) so that the pH value (7.4) is set accordingly.

2.1.2 2,3-Butane-dione-monoxime solution (BDM)

In order to counteract tissue death and autolytic processes after removal of the heart ear, the tissue was stored in a Tyrode solution mixed with BDM (3g/L). Here, too, carbogen is added for buffering to create a stable pH value of 7.4.

BDM serves as cardioplegic protection, as it prevents possible contractions that could be triggered by calcium released during extraction and preparation. BDM is a phosphatase and mediates its effect via reversible inhibition of cross-bridge formation(1) '2. The calcium sensitivity of troponin C and the uptake of calcium into the sarcoplasmic reticulum remain unaffected(3) -4.

Since all effects of BDM are completely reversible by washout, it is an optimal cardioprotective substance for this type of experiment. The exact composition of the buffer and nutrient solutions used is shown in Table 1.

Krebs-Hensele/t buffer			
Cations	**concentration**	***Anions***	**Anion concentration**
Na⁺	152 mmot/L	***Cl⁻***	129.5 mmoVL
K⁺	3.6 mmol/L	$HCO_{(3)}$ $^{(-)}$	25 mmol/L
Mg²⁺	0.6 mmol/L	$H_2PO_{(4)}$ $^{(-)}$	1.3 mmol/L
Ca²⁺	0.2 mmol/L	***$SO_{(4)}$ $^{(2-)}$***	0.6 mmolL
Tyrode solution		*BDM-Tyrode solution*	
Solid	**Weighed sample (1 L)**	***Solid***	**Weighed sample (1 litre)**
NaCl	7.422 g	***NaCl***	7,422 g
$NaHCO_3$	2.100g	***2,3-BDM***	3,000 g

Glucose	2.016g	***$NaHCO_3$***	2,100 g
KH_2PO_4	0.177 g	***glucose***	2.01 fig
KCl	0,172g	***KH_2PO_4***	0,177 g
$MgSO_4$-$7H_2O$	0,146 g	*KCl*	0,172 g
$CaCl_2$-$2H_2O$	0.029 g	***$MgSO_47H_2O$***	0.146 g
Old insulin	5I.U.	***$CaCl_2$-$2H_2O$***	0.029 g

Table 1: Composition of the buffer solutions used

2.2 Atrial tissue

The tissue used in this study was obtained during cardiac surgery. These were mostly aorto-coronary bypass operations, aortic valve replacement operations (AKE) or operations on the ascending aorta (AAE). During these operations, cardiac arrest is induced using a cardioplegic solution that results in a depolarisation block. Beforehand, the patients are connected to the heart-lung machine in order to be able to perform extracorporeal circulation. Venous cannulation is performed via the right atrium as standard. The right atrial appendage (Figure 3) often has to be removed and is thus available for experimental trials.

On average, a preserved heart ear is 2x1x1 cm in size and, depending on its condition, between 2 and 12 trabeculae could be obtained per heart ear.

2.2.1 Preservation and transport

After the surgeon has removed the heart ear, it is placed with sterile forceps in a plastic beaker containing approximately 100 ml of carbogen gassed and cooled (4°C) BDM-Tyrode solution. It is then immediately (10 minutes) taken to the laboratory and preparation can begin. If the experiment cannot be performed immediately, the heart ear should be cooled temporarily.

2.2.2 Preparation

The preparation of the trabeculae carneae (Figure 4) was carried out in a preparation dish filled with cooled and carbogen-saturated BDM tyrode using a stereomicroscope (Olympus, VMT) with 10x magnification. The preparation was carried out with microsurgical instruments (forceps, microscissors of different sizes). It is important to work as atraumatically as possible in order to avoid irreversible damage to the trabeculae. For this reason, the dissected trabeculae were also transferred to a separate container (again with BDM Tyrode) using a plastic pipette to avoid possible damage due to stretching and then immediately cooled again. The trabeculae obtained in this way can then be used for experiments with the strip system at .

In principle, the trabeculae should not have a larger cross-section than 0.64 mm[(2)] (diameter 0.9 mm), as the tissue is supplied exclusively via diffusion due to the fact that there is no longer any blood flow and there is therefore a risk of hypoxia with thicker trabeculae. In addition, trabeculae that are as unbranched as possible and not at the edges are best suited, as these can be dissected out most atraumatically and only need to be cut at the respective ends.

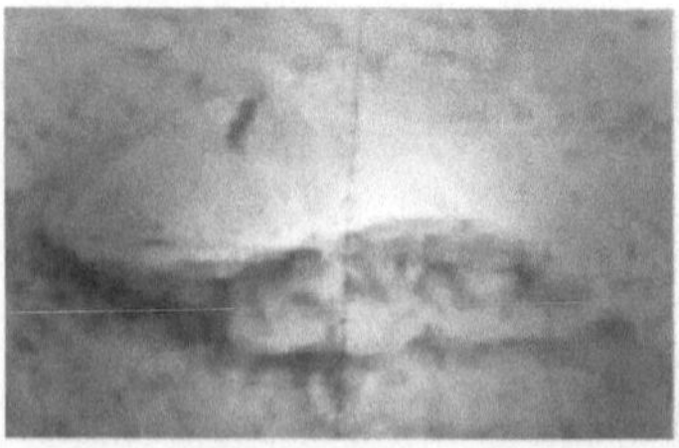

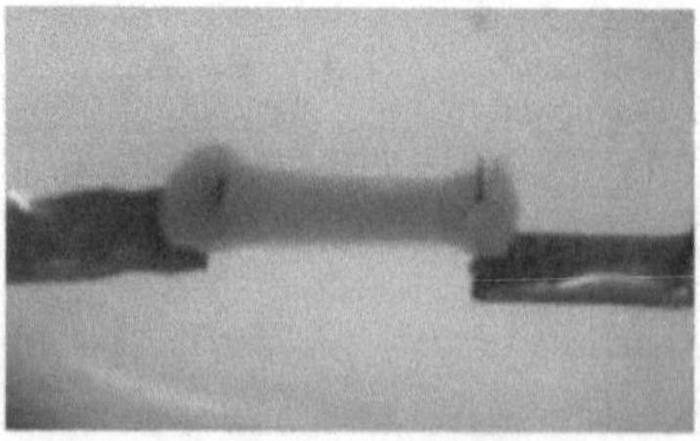

Figure 3: Right heart ear, view through the microscope
Figure 4: Isolated trabecula fixed on needles, view through the microscope

2.2.3 Declaration of consent

For all tissue samples obtained, a declaration of consent was signed by the patients beforehand, which was acquired by the Department of Cardiac Surgery Graz as part of the informed consent process.

A corresponding vote of the ethics committee is available for the experiments carried out (ethics vote 19-109ex07/08).

2.3 Strip system(s)

The experiments were carried out with two different measurement setups, which are briefly described and illustrated below.

2.3.1 Setup 1

This setup, shown in Figs. 5 and 6, was used for the experiments in which concentration-response curves were determined, as the recirculation system ensures that the amount of liquid in the system is as constant as possible. It consists of the following elements:

- Measuring unit with force transducer (Scientific Instruments, Germany)

- Stimulator STM1 (Scientific Instruments, Germany)

- MC MS roller pump (Ismatec, Switzerland)

- VMT stereomicroscope (Olympus, Japan)

- 4-channel thermal recorder Graohtec Linearcorder WR 3320 (Graohtec, Jaoan)

- Computer with Labview software programme

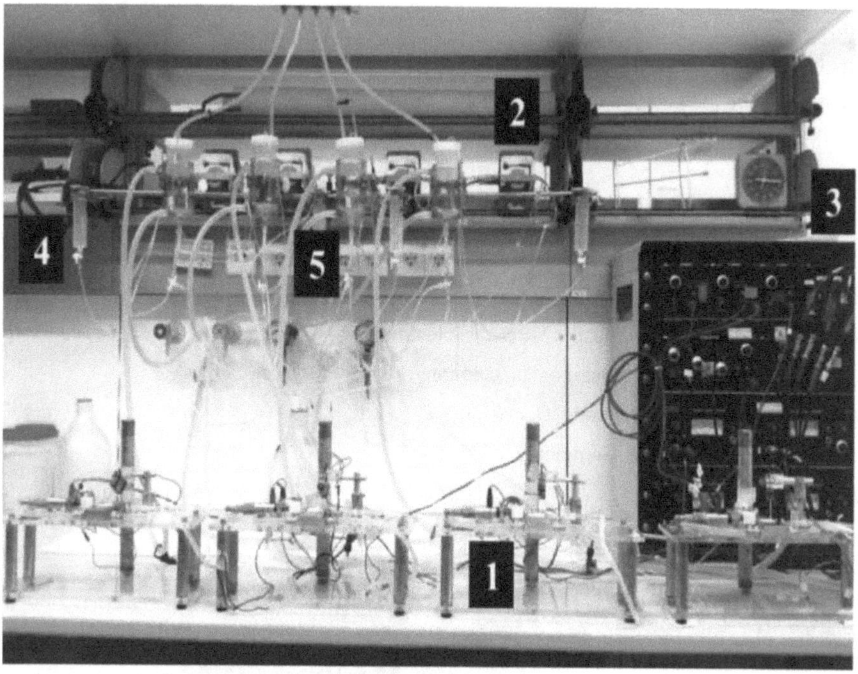

Figure 5: Setup 1, 1: Measuring unit with organ bath, force transducer and micrometer screw, 2: Roller pump, 3: Stimulator, 4: 50 ml perfusor syringe for draining liquid, 5: Tyrode basin with tube system and gassing unit.

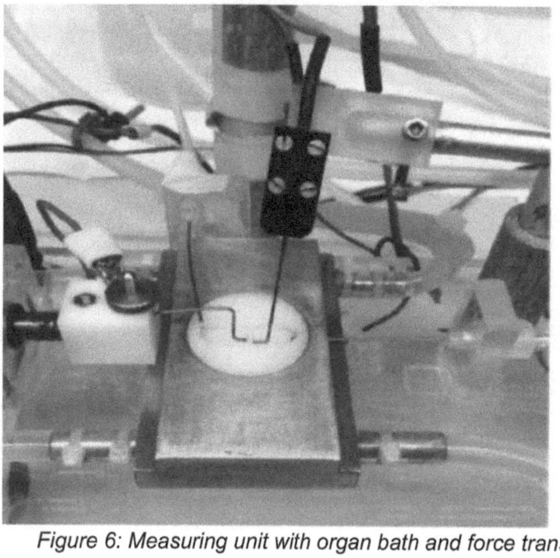

Figure 6: Measuring unit with organ bath and force transducer (black element).

In this setup, the liquid in the organ bath is pumped in via a cannula and sucked out again via another cannula. The liquid is then returned to the Tyrode back to the Tyrode basin. Large sections of the tube system are thermoregulated according to the counterflow principle: The Tyrode circulation system is integrated into the hose system in which the heat pump is embedded, which ensures a constant temperature in the circuit.

2.3.2 Setup 2

This setup, shown in Fig. 7, was used for the experiments in which frequency-dependent effects were determined. It consists of:

- Measuring unit with force transducer (Scientific Instruments, Germany)
- STIM8 stimulator (Scientific Instruments, Germany)
- Thermostat (Scientific Instruments, Germany)
- Stereomicroscope (Optech, Germany)
- A/D converter
- Computer with LabChart software programme

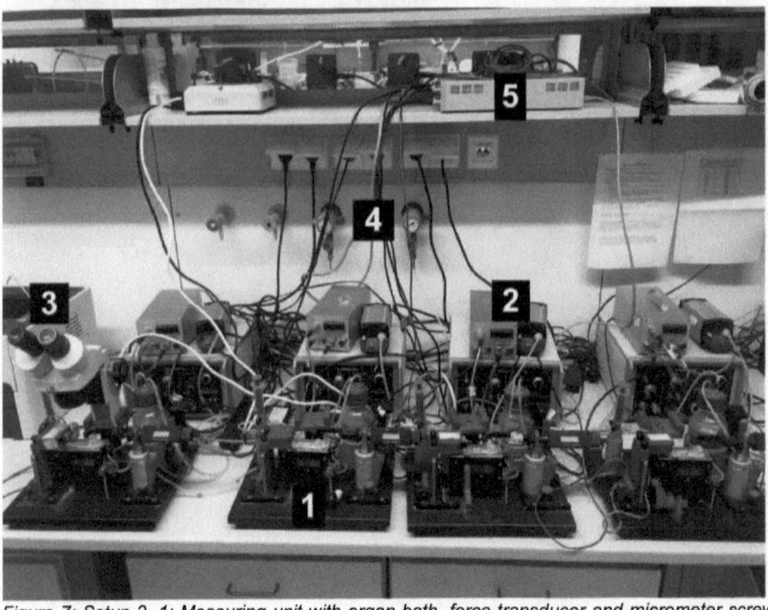

Figure 7: Setup 2, 1: Measuring unit with organ bath, force transducer and micrometer screw, 2: Stimulator and thermostat, 3: Stereomicroscope, 4: Oxygen valve, 5: A/D converter with connection to the computer

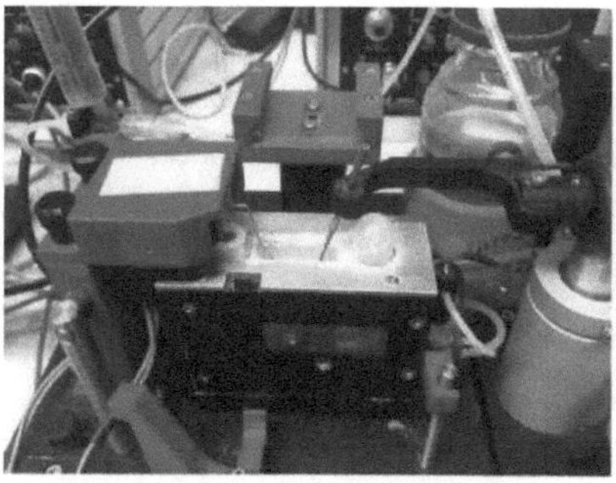

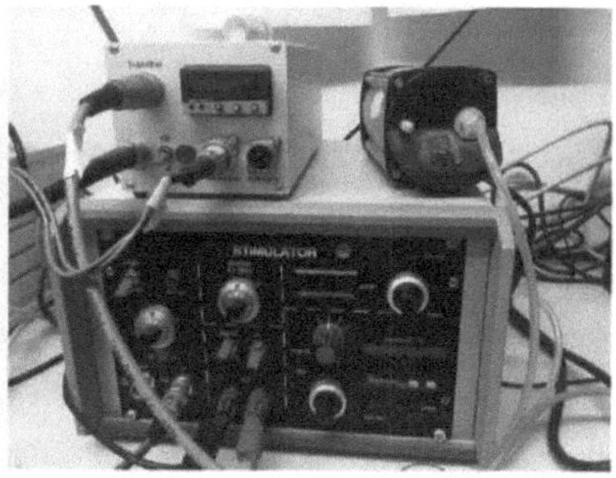

Figure 8: Measuring unit with organ bath and force transducer
Figure 9: Stimulator and thermostat (top)

In contrast to the first setup, this one does not have a circulation system, which is why evaporating liquid could pose a problem during longer experiments. In addition, the arrangement of the stimulators is different here and the stimulation frequencies can be set separately for each channel, which can be advantageous for experiments with different stimulation frequencies. The LabChart computer programme also provides a continuous recording of the entire experiment.

2.4 Experimental procedure

2.4.1 Experimental setup

Both systems described have four channels each, i.e. measurements can be carried out simultaneously with four trabeculae. Each channel has its own organ bath and its own temperature control, which keeps the temperature constant at 37°C. In addition, each channel has its own gassing unit (again with carbogen), which ensures that the circulating substance contains sufficient oxygen and that the pH value remains constant at 7.4.

The organ bath, which forms the central element of the system, is made of Teflon and is enclosed in a thermoblock. The prepared Tyrode solution, to which 2.018 g/l glucose is added as an energy substrate and 5 LE. insulin. One of the two needles on which the trabeculum is suspended is connected to a force transducer that measures the contraction force and kinetic data. This data is then transmitted to a computer with the relevant programme running or, in the case of Setup 1, also to a printer. The other needle is connected to a micrometer screw, which can be used to stretch the trabeculum in a controlled manner. This allows an increasing preload to be simulated and the isometric contraction force increases according to the Frank-Starling mechanism until a maximum value (=Lmax) is reached[5]. Electrical stimulation is provided by a stimulator connected to both needles.

2.4.2 Start of the experiment

After preparation, the trabeculae are attached to the strip system as atraumatically and unstretched as possible using two forceps under the microscope. The BDM tyrode must first be washed out of the trabeculae. This is done in the first setup by draining the first 40 ml of the initially contained 90 ml of Tyrode and removing it from the circuit. This leaves a volume of 50 ml in the system. As this is not possible in the second setup, the trabeculae are washed out in three different plastic beakers filled with Tyrode. The trabeculae are always transferred using a plastic pipette.

After mounting, the respective computer programmes are started and calibrated, after which recording can begin. Before starting the stimulation, a physiological Ca^{2+}concentration must be built up. The first step is to increase the calcium concentration from 0.2 to 1.2 mmol/l by adding 1 mol Ca^{2+}. Then wait about five minutes until the trabeculae have acclimatised to the increased calcium concentration and the stimulation can be started carefully. The concentration can now be increased to 2.5 mmol/l in a further step. In order to avoid an exaggerated reaction to the first calcium step in setup 2, this is divided into three separate steps, as the calcium is absorbed more quickly here due to the lack of a circulatory system.

The stimulation frequency used at the beginning was 1 Hz in all experiments; this was left as it was except in experiments for the force-frequency relationship. The stimulation voltage was usually set between 3 and 6 mV with a pulse duration of 5 ms. The required voltage can vary from trabecula to trabecula. It is usually increased until you see a nice, undeveloped contraction (twitch) and the contraction force no longer changes significantly by further increasing the voltage.

Once everything is set correctly, you can begin to carefully stretch the trabeculae until Lmax is reached. This should be based on how much the diastolic tension increases as a result of the stretching. This should not be more than a third in order to avoid stretching traumas to the trabeculae. Once Lmax has been reached, the actual test protocol can begin.

2.4.3 Freezing and storing the specimens

After the experiment, the trabeculae are removed and transferred to labelled Eppendorf Cryotubes that have been pre-cooled with liquid nitrogen. The sealed tube is then placed directly into a container of liquid nitrogen and placed in a refrigerator (-80°C) at the ZMF Graz for long-term storage.

2.5 Substances

2.5.1 Flecainide

For the flecainide experiments, "Aristocor" ampoules from the cardiological intensive care unit of Graz University Hospital were used. These contain 10 mg/ml flecainide acetate, each ampoule contains 15 ml. Using these ampoules, a stock solution containing $10^{'2}$mol/l flecainide was first prepared with distilled water. A dilution series was then prepared with the required concentrations of 10^{-3}, $10^{-4}$and 10^{-5}mol/l flecainide.

2.5.2 Amiodarone

For the amiodarone experiments, "Sedacoron" ampoules from the cardiological ward of Graz University Hospital were used. These ampoules

contain amiodarone hydrochloride at a concentration of 50 mg/ml in 3 ml of pale yellow liquid. Here too, a stock solution containing 10^{-2} amiodarone was prepared by adding Tyrode and then a dilution series analogous to flecainide was prepared.

2.4.3 Amiodarone solvent

As amiodarone has highly lipophilic properties, it cannot be dissolved in distilled water or Tyrode alone. For this reason, it is also dissolved in 20 mg/ml benzyl alcohol and 10% "Tween 80" (polysorbate 80) in the "Sedacoron" ampoules mentioned above.

In order to recognise and investigate possible cardiotoxic effects caused by the solvent, a mixture of 2% benzyl alcohol, 10% "Tween 80" and 88% distilled water was also prepared for the amiodarone test series. A dilution series with the required concentrations was then prepared in the same way as for flecainide and amiodarone.

2.6 Test protocols

2.6.1 Flecainide concentration-response curve

The purpose of this series of experiments was to investigate the concentration-response curve with regard to the contraction force of flecainide on the human atrial myocardium. After the preparations mentioned in chapter 2.4.2 and reaching a steady state, the cumulative increase of the flecainide concentration can be started. The steps selected were 10^{-8}, 10^{-7}, 10^{-6}, $3*10^{-6}$, $10^{-5}$and IO^mol/l. After each increase in concentration, a wait was made until a steady state was reached again. This time was between 10 and 15 minutes. The same amount of distilled water was added to the control trabeculae. In each experiment, 1-2 intervention and 1-2 control trabeculae from the same heart ear were analysed.

A total of 13 trabeculae and 9 control trabeculae from 9 hearts were analysed to determine the concentration-response curve.

2.6.2 Amiodarone concentration-response curve

The concentration-response curve for amiodarone was determined in the same way as for flecainide. The concentrations selected here were 10^{-8}, 10^{-7}, 10^{-6}, $10^{-5,}10^{-4}$and 10^{-3}mol/l. The time between the individual steps was also 10 to 15 minutes. Since amiodarone is present dissolved in a mixture with benzyl alcohol and "Tween 80" due to its lipophilicity, the control trabeculae were treated with the prepared solvent in order to be able to identify effects mediated by it.

A total of 8 trabeculae with amiodarone and 6 control trabeculae with the solvent from 4 hearts were examined for this series of experiments.

2.6.3 Influence of flecainide on the force-frequency relationship

In order to determine the influence of flecainide on the contraction force as a function of the stimulation frequency, trabeculae were exposed to a concentration of $3*10^{-6}$mol/l flecainide in the organ bath after reaching steady state. The concentration $3*10^{-6}$mol/l was chosen because in another study, in which ventricular myocardium was investigated, this concentration was found to have a half-maximal effect[6]. This also ensures very good comparability of the results.

After the addition of flecainide, 15 minutes were waited until the effect had stabilised and the stimulation frequency was increased from 1.0 to 1.5 - 2.0 - 2.5 and 3 Hz. A steady state was also waited for between the frequency increases. The time required for this was 5 minutes in each case. After reaching 3 Hz, the stimulation frequency was lowered again to 1 Hz in order to be able to observe the reversibility of the effects and whether and to what extent the trabeculae were affected by the high-frequency stimulation.

A total of 8 flecainide trabeculae and 6 control trabeculae from 3 hearts were examined for this protocol.

2.6.4 Influence of amiodarone on the force-frequency relationship

To determine the influence of amiodarone and the solvent on the contraction force as a function of the stimulation frequency, the trabeculae were exposed to a concentration of 10^{-4}mol/l amiodarone or the equivalent dose of solvent. The concentration of 10^{-4}mol/l amiodarone was chosen because it corresponds to the therapeutically effective plasma level as it can be detected as a tissue level in the myocardium[7].

The patient then waited 15 minutes and the stimulation frequency was increased analogue to the protocol described in 2.5.3.

A total of 6 amiodarone-treated and 5 solvent-treated trabeculae from 4 hearts were analysed.

2.7 Patient data

The following tables provide an overview of the patient demographics of the individual test series. The parameters recorded were gender (m/f), age (years ± SD), rhythm (sinus rhythm or VHFA), operation (CABG, AKE, CABG + AKE or AAE) and ejection fraction (EF in % ± SD). The following medication groups were also recorded: Acetylsalicylic acid (T-ASS), β- blockers, ACE inhibitors, angiontensin receptor blockers (ARB), angiotensin + neprilysin receptor blockers (ARB/Nep), diuretics, aldosterone antagonists (Aldosterone-Anta.), calcium blockers (Calcium-Anta.), alpha-blockers and antiarrhythmics.

Flecainide KWK, N=9			
Gender [f/m]	0,22/0,78	**Medication:**	
Age [years]	63,22 ± 12,4	T-ASS	56%
Sinus rhythm [%]	89%	β-blocker	44%
VHFA [%]	11 %	ACE inhibitors	44%
CABG [%]	44%	Diuretics	22%
LFS [%]	22%	Aldosterone-Anta.	11 %
AAE [%]	33%	Calcium-Anta.	22%
EF [%]	55,0 ± 6,22 %	Alpha-blocker	44%

Table 2: Patient demographics of the flecainide CHP experiments

Amiodarone CHP, N=4			
Gender [f/m]	0,25/0,75	**Medication:**	
Age [years]	67,25 ± 8,02	T-ASS	100%
Sinus rhythm [%]	100%	β-blocker	100%
CABG [%]	75%	ACE inhibitors	50%
AKE [%]	25%		
EF [%]	52,63 ± 4,75 %		

Table 3: Patient demographics of the amiodarone CHD experiments

Flecainide CFB, N=3			
Gender [f/m]	0,00/1,00	**Medication:**	
Age [years]	69 ± 5,29	T-ASS	66%
Sinus rhythm [%]	100	β-blocker	33%
CABG [%]	33	ACE inhibitors	66%
CABG + ACE [%]	66	ARB	33%
EF [%]	50,8 ± 2,89 %	Diuretics	66%

Table 4: Patient demographics of the flecainide CFB experiments

Amiodarone CFB, N=4			
Gender [f/m]	0,50/0,50	**Medication:**	
Age [years]	66 ± 9,42	T-ASS	50%
Sinus rhythm [%]	100%	β-blocker	50%
CABG [%]	50%	ACE	25%
AKE [%]	50%	ARB/Nep	25%
EF [%]	49,4 ± 17,37%	Diuretics	25%
		Aldosterone-Anta.	25%

Table 5: Patient demographics of the amiodarone CFB experiments

2.8 Analysis

The data collected in the first setup were recorded with LabView using an average of five consecutive contractions at the respective measurement times. For the data collected with LabChart, a period of 30 to 120 contractions with stable ratios was selected at the measurement times and a mean value was calculated from this.

2.8.1 Parameters analysed

The following parameters were analysed during the experiments:

- Developed force	(mN)	Amplitude of the isometric contraction
- Diastolic tension	(mN)	Resting force/tension of the trabecula
-RT50	(ms)	Time from the time of maximum developed force to 50% relaxation
-RT90	(ms)	Time from the time of maximum developed force to 90% relaxation

The measured force data were normalised to the cross-sectional area of the trabeculae ($mN/mm^{2)}$. The systolic force and the diastolic tension were then expressed as a percentage of the initial value (Agw) for better comparability of trabeculae of different strengths. The baseline value defined here was the measurement time after Lmax was reached, shortly before the respective substance was added for the first time.

2.8.2 Statistical analysis

Two-way repeated measures ANOVA tests were carried out to analyse the results statistically. Sidak's multiple comparisons test was used for comparison between the experimental groups (marked with #) and Dunnett's multiple comparisons test for comparison between the intervention group and the baseline (BL) (marked with *).

Significant results were assumed at values $p < 0.05$ and are marked with an * or a # in the diagrams. In addition, $p < 0.01$ was labelled with **/##, $p < 0.001$ with ***/### and $p < 0.0001$ with ****/#### to highlight highly significant results more clearly.

All results are given as mean values ± standard error (SEM) or graphically with error bars.

CHAPTER 3

Results

3.1 Flecainide concentration-response curve (CHC)

The CHP for flecainide was performed according to the protocol described in the methods section. The concentration range analysed was between $10^{-8}$and 10^{-4}mol/l flecainide at a stimulation frequency of 1 Hz. The values are given as a percentage of the initial value (Agw).

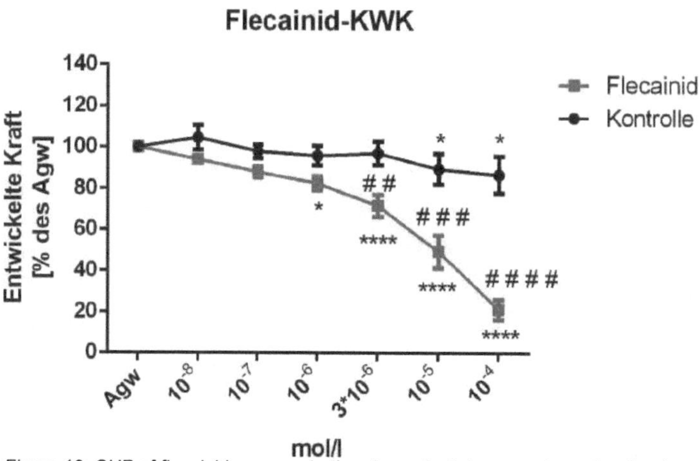

*Figure 10: CHP of flecainide, concentration-dependent decrease in contraction force of flecainide trabeculae (red, n=13) compared to a slight linear decrease in control trabeculae (black, n=9) in per cent of baseline (% Agw + SEM). ##: p<0.01; ###: p<0.001; ####: P<0.0001 to the control group. *: p<0,05; ****: P<0.0001 to baseline (Agw).*

Figure 10 shows a concentration-dependent negative inotropic effect of flecainide. The effect is significant from a concentration of $3x10^{-6}$compared to the control group and increases further with increasing concentration. Overall, the force decreased to 21.16 ± 4.85 % of the initial value.

The slight continuous decrease in the contraction force of the control trabeculae can be attributed to the loss of power ("rundown") of cardiac muscle trabeculae after reaching Lmax. Here, however, the contraction force at the last measurement point was still 86.68 ± 9.02 % of the initial value.

3.1.1 Diastolic tension under flecainide

The course of the diastolic tension shown here in Figure 11 is also not significantly influenced by an increase in the flecainide concentration. Only at 10^{-4}mol/l is there a slight increase in tension compared to the slightly lower values before. However, all changes do not reach the significance level.

In the control trabeculae, the tension tends to decrease slightly (also n.s.).

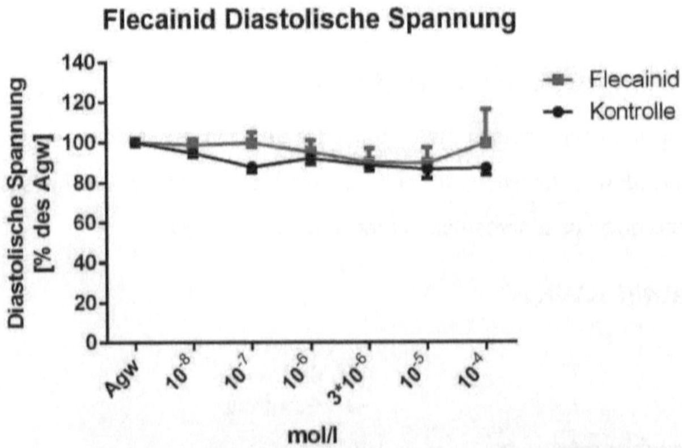

Figure 11: Diastolic tension (% Agw ± SEM) with increasing flecainide concentration of the intervention trabeculae (red) and the control trabeculae (black), overall no significant changes.

3.1.2 Time parameters of isometric relaxation under flecainide

The concentration-dependent influence of flecainide on the time parameters of isometric contraction shown in Figures 12 and 13 is given here in milliseconds (ms). No significant changes occur with flecainide. At most, somewhat similar tendencies to increase, as described above for the diastolic force, are visible.

In the control trabeculae, RT50 and RT90 remain largely constant.

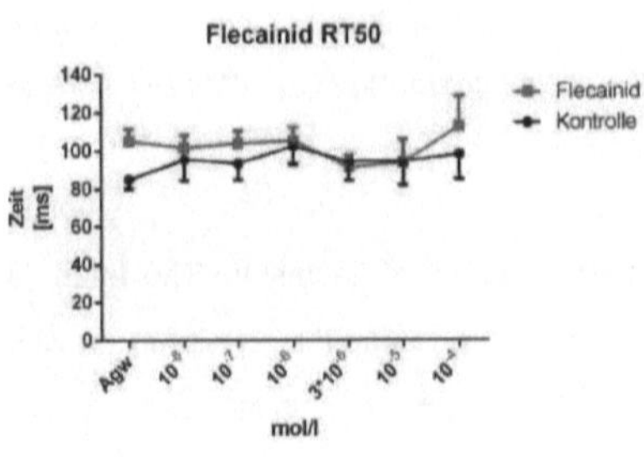

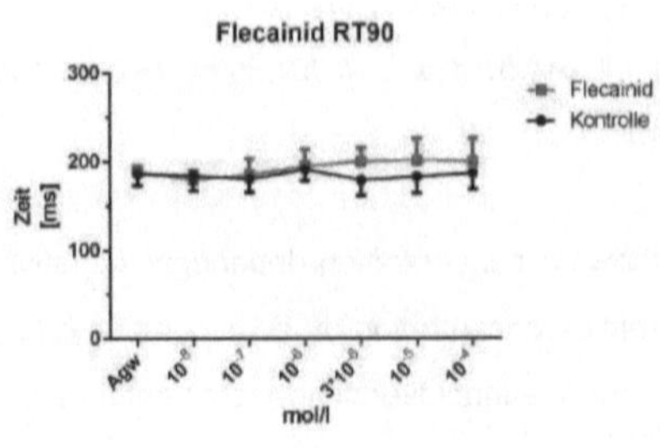

Figure 12: Time parameters of relaxation RT50 (ms ± SEM) with increasing flecainide concentration (left), no significant effect.

Figure 13: Time parameter of relaxation RT90 (ms ± SEM) with increase in flecainide concentration (right), no significant effect.

3.2 Amiodarone concentration-response curve

The CHP for amiodarone (Figure 14) was performed according to the protocol described in the methods section. The concentration range investigated was from $10^{-8}$to 10^{-3}mol/l amiodarone or the equivalent dose of solvent applied cumulatively. This made it possible to discriminatively identify the inotropic effects of amiodarone and those attributable to the solvent.

As Figure 14 shows, there was a clear negative inotropic effect both under the influence of amiodarone and when the solvent was applied. At the maximum concentration of 10^{-3}mol/l, the developed force of amiodarone is reduced to 26.14 ± 5.14 % and of the solvent to 18.50 ± 8.55 %. The values are again given as a function of the initial value. The effect is concentration-dependent and differs significantly from the initial value from 10^{-5}mol/l for amiodarone and from 10^{-4}mol/l for the solvent. The curves diverge in the middle range with a clearly greater decrease in force in the amiodarone group, which reaches the significance level at a concentration of 10^{-5}mol/l. A substance-specific negative inotropic effect of amiodarone (over and above that of the solvent) can therefore be demonstrated in this concentration range.

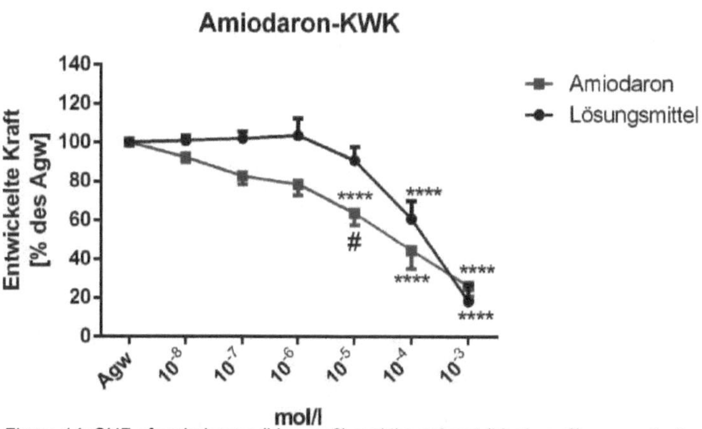

*Figure 14: CHP of amiodarone (blue, n=8) and the solvent (black, n=6), concentration-dependent decrease in contraction force as a percentage of the initial value (% Agw + SEM) in both groups. #: p<0.05 between the groups. ****: p<0.0001 from baseline.*

3.2.1 Diastolic tension under amiodarone

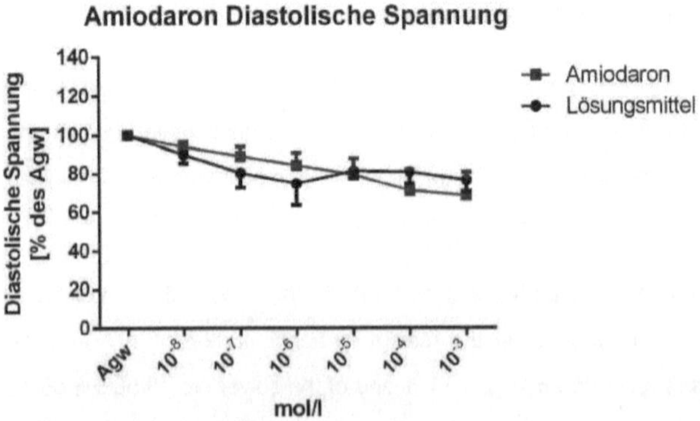

Figure 15: Diastolic tension (% Agw ± SEM) with increase in amiodarone (blue) and solvent concentration (black), slight decrease in tension in both groups (n.s.).

The diastolic tension (Figure 15) shows a very similar course under amiodarone and the solvent. The voltage decreases slightly in both curves during the course of the experiment, but the decrease is not significant. For amiodarone, the voltage at 10'^{3}mol/l is 68.50 ± 12.28 % and for the solvent 76.60 ± 6.02 % of the initial value.

3.2.2 Time parameters of isometric relaxation under amiodarone

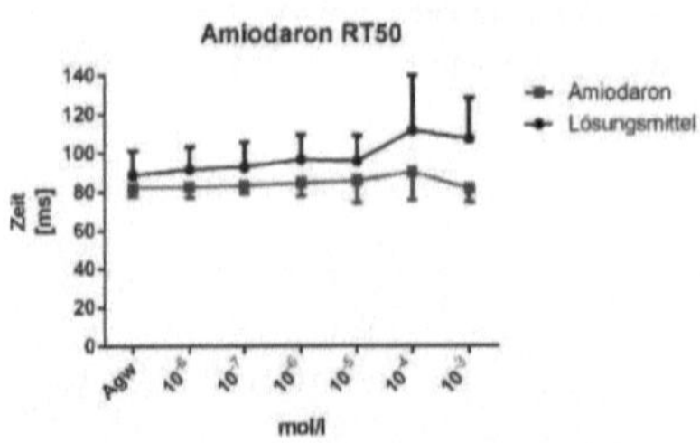

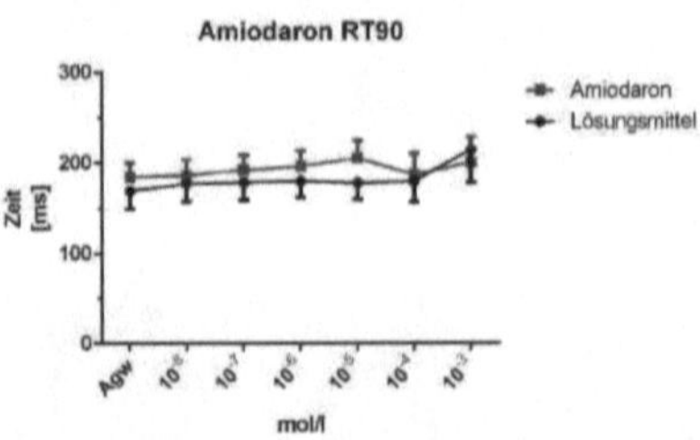

Figure 16: Time parameters of relaxation RT50 (ms + SEM) with increasing amiodarone or solvent concentration (left), no significant effect.

Figure 17: Time parameter of relaxation RT90 (ms ± SEM) with increase in amiodarone or solvent concentration (right), slight increase in RT90 at 10~^{3}mol/l (n.s.).

The relaxation times RT50 and RT90 shown in Figures 16 and 17 do not change significantly with increasing amiodarone concentration, and no clear tendency in one direction is recognisable.

The same applies to the trabeculae treated with solvent. Although there is a slight increase in the RT90 at 10'^{3}mol/l, this is not significant. The RT50 remains largely unchanged even at this concentration.

3.3 Flecainide force-frequency relationship

The force-frequency relationship for flecainide was determined with the concentration 3*10'^6mol/l flecainide. As controls, trabeculae were again exposed to the same equivalent amount of distilled water as would be required at the corresponding flecainide concentration.

The frequency range investigated was 1 Hz to 3 Hz or 60 to 180 bpm. As explained in the methods section, the substance was added first and after a 15-minute waiting period the stimulation frequency was increased by half a Hz in 5-minute increments.

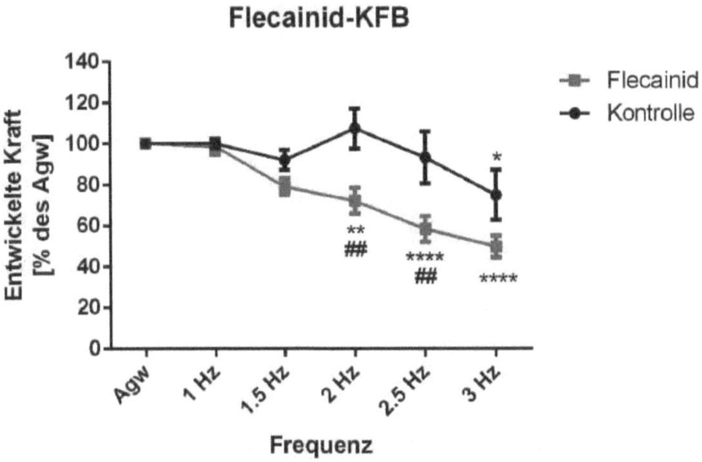

*Figure 18: Course of the force-frequency relationship of flecainide (red, n=8) for the concentration 3*10"6mol/l in per cent of the initial value (% Agw ± SEM); the control trabeculae (black, n=6) show a discreetly positive KFB, while it becomes negative throughout under flecainide. ##: p<0.01 to the control group. *: p<0.05; **: p<0.01; ****; p<0.0001 to the Agw.*

As can be seen in Figure 18, the control trabeculae have their optimum frequency at 2 Hz, with a subtle average increase in force to 107.41 ± 9.81 % compared to the initial value at 1 Hz. Thereafter, the force gradually decreases and reaches its minimum at 3 Hz with 74.90 ± 12.11 %.

Under flecainide, the KFB changes significantly. The developed force decreases continuously with increasing stimulation frequency and reaches its minimum at 3 Hz with 49.77 ± 5.33 % in comparison to the initial value. The differences are significant from 2 Hz compared to both the control trabeculae and the baseline value.

3.3.1 Diastolic tension during flecainide CFB

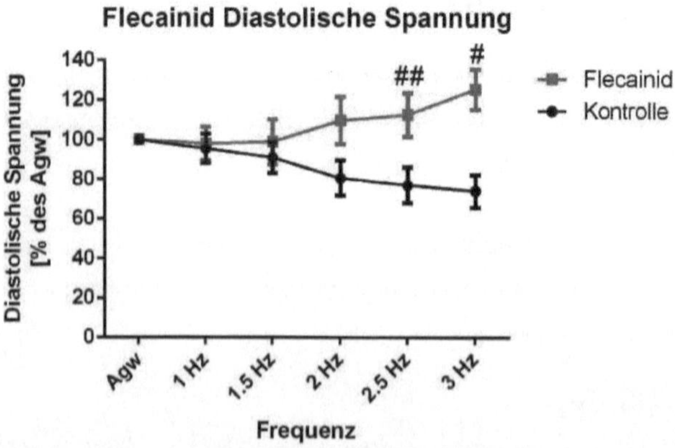

*Figure 19: Course of diastolic tension (% Agw ± SEM) during CFB for the concentration 3*1 Cr^{6}mol/l flecainide, the trabeculae treated with flecainide (red) show a significant increase in diastolic tension compared to the control trabeculae (black) where it decreases slightly. #: $p<0.05$; ##: $p<0.01$ to the control group.*

The diastolic tension also shows a significantly different course between control and flecainide trabeculae, as can be seen here in Figure 19. While the diastolic tension decreases in the control trabeculae and reaches a minimum at 3 Hz with 74.93 ± 9.49 %, it increases in the flecainide trabeculae and reaches its maximum at 3 Hz (125.23 ± 10.08 % of Agw).

3.3.2 Time parameters of isometric relaxation during flecainide CFB

The time parameters of isometric relaxation RT50 and RT90 shorten equally in both groups with increasing stimulation frequency for both the control and the flecainide trabeculae (Figures 20 and 21). The values of the treated group tend to be higher for both time parameters than those of the control group (n.s.).

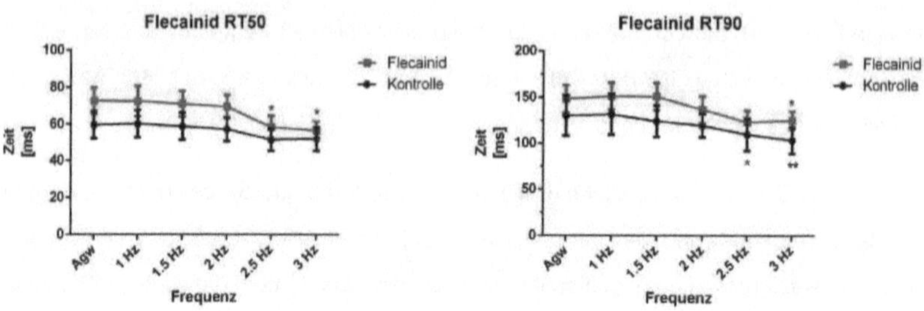

Figure 20: Course of the RT50 (ms ± SEM) during KFB for the concentration 3 10T^{6}mol/l flecainide (left), showing a shortening of the relaxation times from 2.5 Hz. *: $p<0.05$ to the Agw.*

*Figure 21: Course of the RT90 (ms ± SEM) during the KFB for the concentration 3*1 Or⁶mol/l flecainide (right), showing a shortening of the relaxation times from 2.5 Hz. *: p<0.05; **: p<0.01 to the Agw.*

3.3.3 Frequency dependence of the flecainide effects

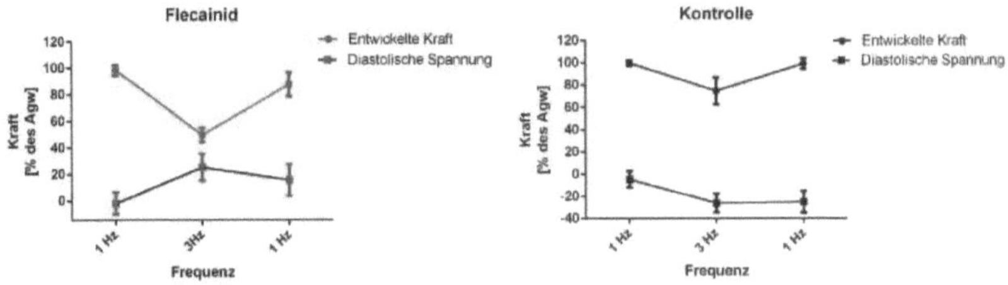

*Figure 22: Effects of 3*10^(-) (6)mol/l flecainide before, during and after CFB (red), the reduced force at 3 Hz almost returns to its initial value at 1 Hz after switching to 1 Hz and the increased diastolic tension also decreases again. Figure 23: Effects of CFB on the control trabeculae (black) before, during and after the intervention, the reduced force at 3 Hz builds up again to its level at 1 Hz, but the reduced diastolic tension remains even after the intervention.*

After reaching 3 Hz, the stimulation frequency was reduced back to 1 Hz to test the extent to which the effects of flecainide were only time-dependent or actually frequency-dependent. Switching to the initial frequency showed a reversibility of the effects and thus proof of a clear frequency-dependent effect (Figure 22).

In the control group, the trabeculae returned to their original level at 1 Hz with a force of 99.30 ± 4.53 %. The diastolic tension remained reduced at 74.93 ± 9.49 %.
In the flecainide group, the effects were also largely reversible and the trabeculae regained a force of 87.91 ± 8.98 % compared to 49.77 ± 5.33 % at 3 Hz. The built-up diastolic tension also decreases again slightly to 115.52 ± 11.77%.

3.4 Amiodarone force-frequency relationship

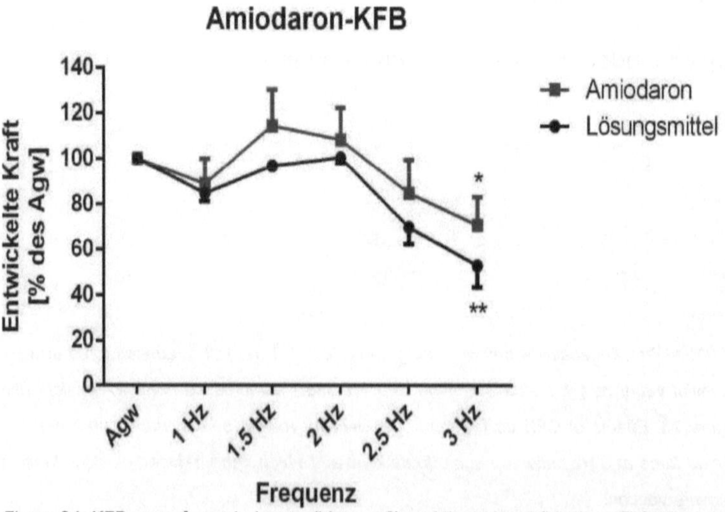

*Figure 24: KFB curve for amiodarone (blue, n=6) and the solvent (black, n=5) for the concentration 10⁴mol/l, both groups show a positive KFB, a decrease in force only occurs from 2.5 Hz. *: p<0.05; **: p<0.01 to the Agw.*

The KFB determined at a concentration of 10^{-4}mol/l does not change significantly between amiodarone and the solvent (Figure 24). Both curves initially show a positive force curve, which then only decreases at higher frequencies of 2.5 and 3 Hz.

Under amiodarone, the trabeculae had their optimum frequency at 1.5 Hz with a maximum of 114.41 ± 16.06 % compared to the initial value and then decreased to a minimum of 70.78 ± 12.27 at 3 Hz.For the control trabeculae treated only with solvent, after an initial drop to 84.77 ± 3.50 % at 1 Hz, their maximum was at 2 Hz with 100.55 ± 2.55 % compared to the initial value. They also had their minimum at 3 Hz with 52.96 ± 9.58 %.

3.4.1 Diastolic tension during amiodarone CFB

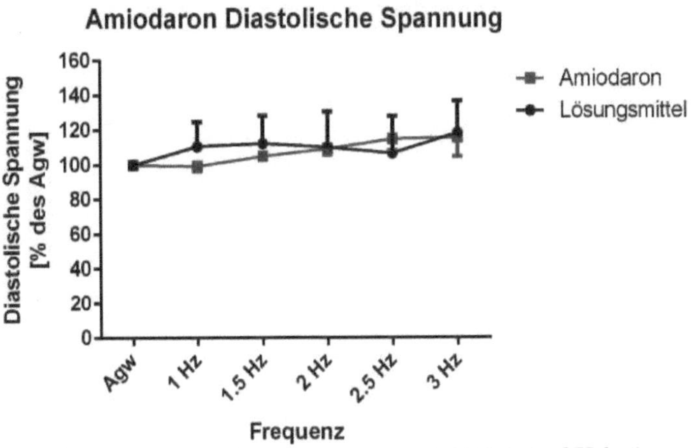

Figure 25: Progression of diastolic tension (% Agw ± SEM) during CFB for the concentration $10^{(-)\,(4)}$mol/l amiodarone or the solvent equivalent, the tension continuously increases slightly in both groups (n.s.).

For the diastolic tension, the amiodarone and solvent trabeculae show a similar course and tend to show a slight continuous increase to a maximum of 115.77 ± 10.88 % for amiodarone and 118.35 ± 18.51 % for the solvent at 3 Hz (Figure 25).

3.4.2 Time parameters of isometric relaxation during amiodarone CFB

The time parameters of isometric contraction shown here for amiodarone and the solvent (Figures 26 and 27), RT50 and RT90, remain largely constant even with increasing stimulation frequency. Only at 3 Hz is there a shortening of the RT90 in both groups. Overall, the effects are similar to those of the flecainide and control groups (Chapter 3.3.2).

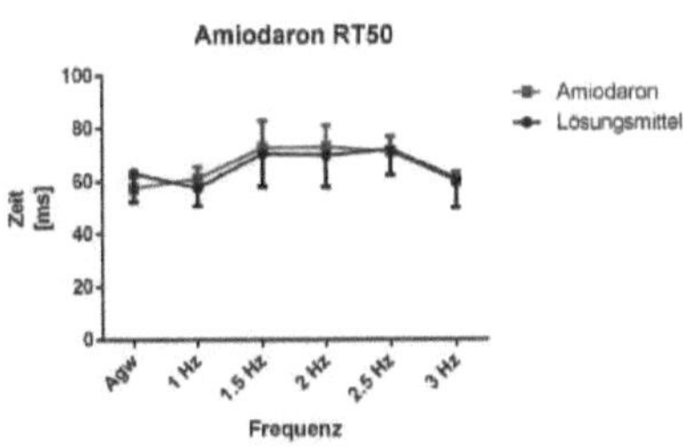

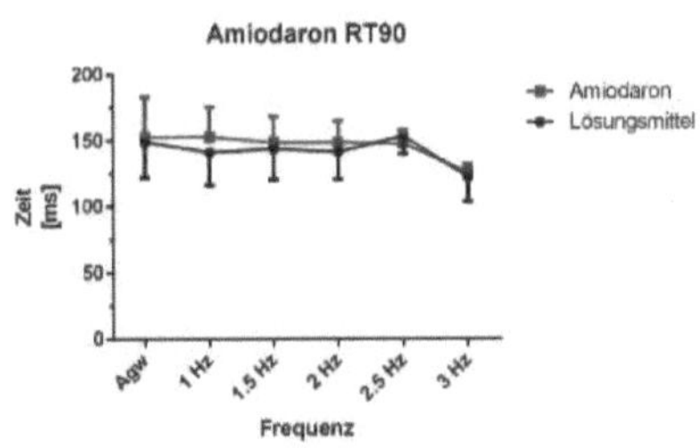

Figure 26: Course of the RT50 (ms ± SEM) during CFB for the concentration 10^{-4}mol/l amiodarone or solvent (left), no significant effect.

Figure 27: Course of the RT90 (ms ± SEM) during the CFB for the concentration $10^{(-)\,(4)}$mol/l amiodarone or solvent (right), there is a shortening of the RT90 at 3 Hz (n.s.).

3.4.3 Frequency dependence of the amiodarone Z-solvent effects

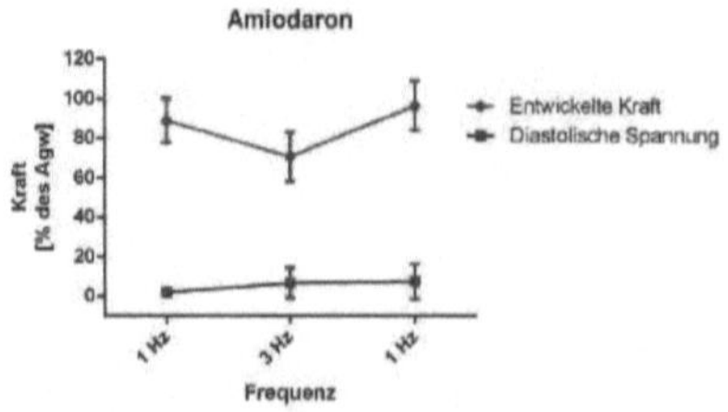

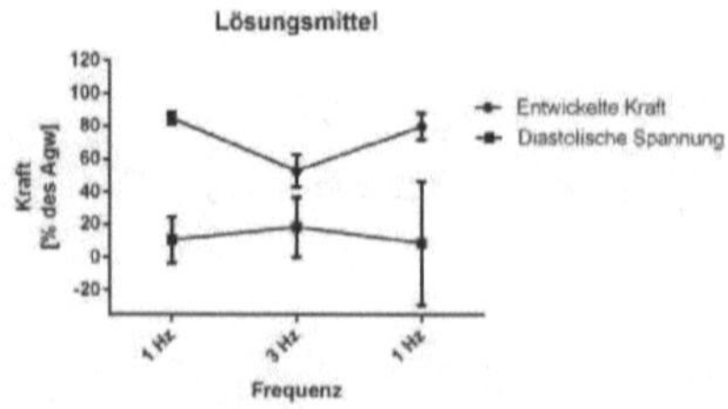

Figure 28: Effects of $10^{(-)\,(4)}$mol/l amiodarone before, during and after CFB (blue), the reduced force at 3 Hz builds up again after the intervention even more than its original level at 1 Hz, but the increased diastolic tension remains approximately at this level even at 1 Hz.

Figure 29: Effects of the solvent equivalent of $10^{(-)\,(4)}$mol/l amiodarone before, during and after CFB (black), the reduced force at 3 Hz builds up again almost to its original level at 1 Hz, the slightly increased diastolic tension decreases again after the intervention.

Here, too, the stimulation frequency was reduced to 1 Hz after reaching 3 Hz in order to measure the effects that occurred.

In the amiodarone group, the trabeculae reached a force of 96.46 ± 12.41 %, even more than their original level at 1 Hz of 88.82 ± 11.15 %. This characterises the decrease in force as purely frequency-related. The diastolic tension, on the other hand, does not react purely frequency-dependent, but continues to increase slightly, which speaks in favour of a time-dependent effect of amiodarone on the diastolic tension.

In the solvent group, the effects on both contraction force and diastolic tension are largely reversible. After a change in frequency, the trabeculae regain a force at a level similar to that at the initial frequency of 1 Hz. The built-up diastolic tension also decreases again after its increase at 3 Hz.

CHAPTER 4

Discussion

In this study, the effects of flecainide and amiodarone on human atrial multicellular myocardial strips were investigated for the first time. It was shown that flecainide mediates a concentration-dependent negative inotropic effect and also negatively alters the force-frequency relationship (CFR) of the heart. Amiodarone and its solvent also showed a concentration-dependent negative inotropic effect, with the solvent itself having the strongest effects at high concentrations. The CFB was not significantly altered in either the amiodarone or the solvent group.

4.1 Inotropic effects and mechanism of action of flecainide

In the experiments performed, a concentration-dependent negative inotropic effect on the atrial myocardium could be demonstrated for flecainide, which shows its half-maximal effect (ECso) at a concentration of approx. $7*10^{-6}$mol/l flecainide. These results are consistent with the findings of other authors. Schulze and Knops were able to demonstrate this dose-dependent negative inotropic effect in ventricular trabeculae from calves[30], Ito et al. in isolated trabeculae from rabbit and rat hearts[31]and C. Pagel in trabeculae from rabbit hearts and insufficient human ventricular trabeculae[6].

Flecainide as a class Ic antiarrhythmic agent exerts its effect primarily by inhibiting fast voltage-dependent Na^+ channels, which are responsible for the initiation of the action potential. This prolongs phase 0 of the action potential and the relative refractory period, which can suppress incoming extrasystoles. By performing rapid cooling contractures (RCC), which can be used to infer the Ca^{2+}content of the SR, Ito et al. were able to show that blocking the Na^+ channel and the associated reduced Na^+ influx into the cell also reduces the stored Ca^{2+}in the SR. In line with this, a visible measurable signal of the intracellular calcium transient was generated in the work of C. Pagel using aequorin, thus demonstrating the calcium dependence of the negative inotropic effect[6].

4.1.1 Flecainide effects on direct Ca^{2+}regulators (NCX, LTCC, SERCA)

One possible mechanism of the inotropic effect is due to increased Ca^{2+}export from the cell by the sodium-calcium exchanger (NCX), which is stimulated by the increased sodium gradient[31]. It can therefore be assumed that flecainide increases the activity of the NCX.

For flecainide, a blockade of the L-type sarcolemmal calcium channel (LTCC) was also demonstrated by Scamps et al. in frog myocardium[37], Kihara et al. in dog myocardium[38]and Yamashita et al. in rabbit myocardium[(43)]. This could also explain or contribute to the negative inotropic effect. However, the exact plasma concentration above which this effect becomes relevant in vivo is unclear. In the experiments, the effect on the LTCC was shown at concentrations > 10^{-5}mol/L. The therapeutic range for arrhythmias is between $4*10^{-7}$mol/l and $2*10^{-6}$mol/l (200-1000 ng/ml)[39], whereby the lower limit should be used to avoid dangerous side effects such as ventricular arrhythmias. Therefore, possible effects due to the inhibition of LTCC probably play a subordinate role in practice. However, in the experiments conducted as part of this work, inhibition of the LTCC at the higher flecainide concentrations, at which the negative inotropic effect was very pronounced, could play a role.

In addition, Bisping et al. were also able to demonstrate direct inhibition of SERCA by flecainide, presumably via the regulatory protein phospholamban (PLB), which also explains a calcium-dependent negative inotropic effect[69]. This could also explain the previously unknown mechanism of action of flecainide in CPVT, as Bai et al. found in PLB-deficient knockout mice, which also carried the CPVT gene, that the elimination of PLB effectively suppressed the arrhythmias[73].

4.1.2 Flecainide effects on K^+ channels

Several studies have also shown that flecainide also has a blocking effect on K^+ channels. Yue et al. were able to demonstrate a blocking

effect on the kur in dog myocytes[42], Yamashita et al. demonstrated a blocking effect on the outwardly rectifying Ito in rabbit myocytes[43]and Wang et al. demonstrated a blocking effect on the Ito but not on the IKUP in human atrial myocytes[44]. In a more recent study, Melgari et al. were also able to demonstrate the effect of flecainide on human Nr at therapeutic plasma levels (EC50 = $1.5*10^{-6}$mol/l) and shed further light on the molecular basis of this[41]. This is consistent with an observed prolonged APD[45], as well as with possible QT time prolongations, which is why additional caution is required here if there is a risk of long QT syndrome (LQTS)[41]. Overall, the antiarrhythmic effect of flecainide therefore appears to be influenced not only by blockade of Na, but also by blockade of Nr. However, the extent to which this also influences inotropic effects and the force-frequency relationship is unclear.

4.1.3 Flecainide and the ryanodine receptor

The effect of flecainide on the ryanodine receptor RyR2[36]located on the sarcoplasmic reticulum has been controversially discussed in recent years, which could also result in inotropic effects. This was prompted by a publication by Watanabe et al. in which the efficacy of flecainide in catecholaminergic polymorphic ventricular tachycardia (CPVT) was established using a mouse model and in female patients[32]. CPVT is caused by a mutation of RyR2, which can lead to partially uncontrolled Ca^{2+}release from the SR, which can subsequently trigger potentially fatal ventricular tachycardia. Thus, the initial data suggested a direct effect of flecainide on RyR2[32]. Hilliard et al. were able to substantiate this with further experiments using isolated myocytes from mice and rats[33]. However, in subsequent studies, including those by Bannister et al, who worked with voltage clamp techniques, this mechanism of action could not be confirmed. They explained the effect rather by secondary effects caused by the known Na^+ -channel blockade of flecainide. For example, by the reduced intracellular Ca^{2+}concentration described above through activation of the NCX, as a result of the reduced cytosolic Na^+ concentration, and the resulting possibly reduced stimulus threshold to trigger an action potential[3435]. Therefore, RyR2 does not appear to play a role in the negative inotropic effects described here.

4.2 Influence of flecainide on the force-frequency relationship

This study also demonstrated a flecainide-altered split KFB in human atrial myocardium. Here, 1 Hz was chosen as the initial frequency, as this represents a more physiological value in contrast to the 0.5 Hz used in many other studies. The concentration $3*10^{-6}$was chosen for the experiments, as this was calculated as EC50 in another study with ventricular myocardium[6]. In addition, the value is at the upper end of the therapeutic plasma concentration[39]in order to have the best possible practical relevance and at the same time to be able to visualise effects as well as possible. The CFB performed in this way was weakly positive for the controls, with a maximum increase in force to around 110% of the initial value at 2 Hz, but the force then decreased again with increasing stimulation frequency. In contrast, the KFB for the flecainide trabeculae was completely negative and decreased to 50% of the initial value at 3 Hz.

C. Pagel came to similar results when he examined insufficient human myocardium and healthy rabbit myocardium. The insufficient human myocardium also showed a negative CFB and the CFB of the rabbit myocardium was significantly worsened. Apart from this, they were able to observe not only impaired systolic function, but also impaired diastolic function in both tissues[6]. Ito et al. also showed an almost abolished CFB in rabbit myocardium and a negative CFB in rat myocardium[31]. When making comparisons with other studies, it should be noted that both the origin (atrial or ventricular) and the condition (tissue from insufficient or healthy hearts) of the examined myocardium play a significant role in the CFB. This was shown in a study by Schwinger et al. In contrast to ventricular tissue, the increase in force from 0.5 Hz to 1 Hz (i.e. in a physiologically low range) appears to be by far the most pronounced for atrial tissue. The subsequent decrease in force at higher stimulation frequencies also appears to be more pronounced in atrial tissue than in ventricular tissue[46].

The shown deterioration of CFB by flecainide could be explained by its binding kinetics. As a class I antiarrhythmic agent, flecainide primarily blocks the fast voltage-dependent Na^+ channels (Na) and thus reduces the Na^+ influx into the cell. As has already been shown, a reduced cytosolic Na^+ concentration also appears to lead to a reduced intracellular Ca^{2+}concentration, which subsequently affects the force of contraction[31]. The binding of flecainide to the Na^+ channel depends on its state of activity. It has a high affinity for open and inactivated Na^+ channels, but not when the channel is in a resting state. In addition, flecainide also acts from the cytosolic side, but it must first enter the cell. This is also only possible through open Na^+ channels. The effect of the antiarrhythmic drug is therefore stronger the more often the channel is active per unit of time[3447]. This mechanism of action is also known as "use-dependent block" and could explain why the negative inotropic effects are potentiated at higher stimulation frequencies.

4.3 Diastolic function under flecainide

A further aim of this study was to investigate the effects of flecainide on diastolic function. With constant stimulation at 1 Hz, no clear indication of an influence on diastolic function could be found, even at high concentrations of 10^{-4}mol/l. However, in the experiments, no effect on diastolic function was found for flecainide. However, a significant increase in diastolic tension was recorded in the experiments for the CFB with increasing stimulation frequency. However, the relaxation times of the isometric contraction remained largely unchanged.

This is in line with the present study by C. Pagel, as a frequency-dependent increase in diastolic tension was also shown in both insufficient human ventricular myocardium and in healthy rabbit myocardium. In ventricular myocardium with insufficiency, the concentration-dependent induction of increased diastolic tension and an increase in RT90 was also demonstrated, although this only occurred at high doses (10^{-4}mol/l)[6]. The differences in the concentration-dependent induced effect could be due to the fact that a certain diastolic dysfunction was probably already present in the insufficient myocardium used by C. Pagel. Nevertheless, both studies were able to show that even without pre-existing diastolic dysfunction, flecainide can induce these effects, at least under experimental conditions.

The two mechanisms responsible for Ca^{2+}elimination from the cytosol and thus also for diastolic function are the activities of the sodium-calcium exchanger (NCX) and those of the calcium pump SERCA. Since flecainide indirectly increases the activity of the NCX by reducing Na^+ influx, the diastolic dysfunction caused in these experiments could be due to inhibition of SERCA activity. Inhibition of SERCA activity would also explain the deterioration in CFB, as the increase in SERCA activity at higher frequencies is also more relevant than NCX activity[14]. Bisping et al. were able to demonstrate reduced SERCA activity using a radioactive Ca^{2+}uptake assay and identified the regulatory protein phospholamban as a probable target using Western blotting[69].

4.4 Inotropic effects and mechanism of action of amiodarone and solvents

In the present study, the effects of amiodarone on the non-insufficient atrial myocardium were investigated. In order to differentiate the effects of amiodarone from those of its solvent, parallel controls were performed with its solvent at the same dose as amiodarone. The result was that at a constant stimulation frequency of 1 Hz, both groups showed a very similar, although not exactly the same, concentration-dependent negative inotropic effect. In the medium concentration range from $10^{-7}$to 10^{-4}mol/l the two curves diverged, which was also significant at 10^{-5}mol/l. Amiodarone thus showed a substance-specific negative inotropic effect in this concentration range that went beyond the effect of the solvent. At high concentrations, however, the effect of the solvent itself dominated. At the highest concentration of 10^{-3}mol/l, the effect was even more pronounced in the solvent group than with amiodarone in solvent. C. Pagel also showed a concentration-dependent negative inotropic effect when he compared the effects of amiodarone with those of the solvent in insufficient ventricular myocardium[6]. In C. Pagel's study, however, the amiodarone and solvent groups were virtually identical. These differences could be explained by a selectivity of atrial Na^+ channels of amiodarone[55 68], which could subsequently mediate a negative inotropic effect via secondary Ca^{2+}losses[31]. At higher concentrations, the more pronounced effect of the solvent could then predominate.

The effects shown are consistent with clinical observations initially observed after bolus administration of amiodarone in vivo. These usually show a reduction in LVEF and arterial blood pressure, accompanied by a reactive increase in heart rate[54]. This is one reason why bolus administration of amiodarone is avoided in the clinical setting and it is administered as a short infusion or infusion. These initially observed effects could also be due to the solvent, as its half-life in the blood is only a few minutes[53]and these effects usually disappear again in vivo within 10 minutes. Under the experimental conditions of the tests carried out here, no enzymes responsible for the degradation were present in the organ bath. Another argument in favour of a solvent-mediated effect is that no haemodynamically relevant effects occur when taken orally, apart from a moderate reduction in heart rate thanks to its anti-adrenergic active component[54].

4.4.1 Molecular targets of amiodarone

Amiodarone, although categorised as a class-III antiarrhythmic drug, is actually a multi-channel blocker. However, it exerts its main effect by blocking the K^+ channels and thereby blocks the "delayed rectifier current" (I_K) with the channels kr, I_{KS} and I_{KI}, as well as the K^+ -specific channel Ito. This prolongs the repolarisation (phase 3) of the action potential, the action potential duration (APD) and the absolute refractory period. On the ECG, this can manifest itself in a prolongation of the QT time[(48) -50]. Amiodarone also causes a "use-dependent" inhibition of the fast voltage-dependent Na^+ channel (iNa)[56]. Amiodarone has also been shown to be atrial selective in inhibiting Na in rabbit cardiomyocytes[55]and dog myocardium[68], which, if true in humans, may explain its good efficacy in atrial arrhythmias without affecting ventricular function. Its inhibitory effect on Ca^{2+}channels has also been demonstrated, which also appears to be "use-dependent"[57 58]. Finally, amiodarone also has an anti-adrenergic component. Due to its structural similarity to thyroid hormones, it appears to mediate this via the thyroid hormone receptor (TR) by downregulating ß-receptors[5960]. All these effects may explain the negative inotropic effect of amiodarone observed in the medium concentration range. Another explanation would be a possible influence on the NCX. However, there is contradictory information on this in the literature[(70)'71].

4.4.2 Effects of the solvent

The following factors appear to be relevant for the dominant solvent effect at high concentrations: Intravenous amiodarone is mixed with polysorbate 80 and benzyl alcohol as solubilisers in its standard galenic formulation used in practice . Polysorbate 80 (polyoxyethylene (20) sorbitan monooleate) is an emulsifier and one of the few surface-active substances that are also parenterally compatible. It is found in many foods and medical products and is considered harmless to health. However, there are indications that polysorbate 80 is responsible for the arterial hypotension that occurs after amiodarone bolus injection. Munoz et al. compared the normal formulation of amiodarone with an experimental formulation without polysorbate 80 in patients undergoing coronary angiography with regard to haemodynamic parameters. In contrast to the normal formulation, there was only a very small effect on arterial blood pressure. However, the two groups were identical again after 30 minutes with regard to their haemodynamic and cardiac parameters[61]. Platou et al. were able to show in dogs that solvent alone mediates the same hypotensive effects as amiodarone, but not the electrophysiological effects[62]. Somberg et al. tested a new compound called Amio-Aqueus in rats and found that it showed significantly less hypotensive and cardiodepressive properties[63]. In a more recent study, Lindquist et al. tested a compound containing the sulfoalkyl ether cyclodextrin as a solubiliser on patients during an 18-hour loading regime and found a significant difference in the frequency of hypotension[64].

Effects mediated by benzyl alcohol are also conceivable, as benzyl alcohol as a local anaesthetic also blocks Na^+ channels. In addition, a negative inotropic effect on rabbit myocardium has been described[65]and in Chapter 4.1 it was explained how a reduced Na^+ influx can result in a negative inotropic effect via secondary Ca^{2+}loss through the NCX[31].

4.5 Influence of amiodarone and solvent on the force-frequency relationship

The influence of amiodarone and its solvent on the force-frequency relationship was also investigated in the experiments conducted as part of this work. The concentration used was 10^{-4}mol/l and the frequency range investigated was also from 1 Hz to 3 Hz. The concentration of 10^{-4}mol/l was chosen because this concentration also corresponds to the concentration measured in the myocardium[7]. In contrast to the previously mentioned in-vivo studies on haemodynamics, it can be assumed here that only the acute effects of amiodarone were determined due to the experimental set-up. The same applies to the solvent group, as the enzymes responsible for the enzymatic degradation are not included in the tyrode used here.

The developed force and the course of the KFB did not change significantly between the two groups. Overall, the silhouettes of the curves were similar in shape and progression. In principle, they are also comparable with the curve of the control group from the flecainide experiments. The frequency-dependent increase in force even tended to be highest in the amiodarone-treated group, which therefore completely rules out a deterioration of the CFB. This study was the first to show that amiodarone has no negative effects on the force-frequency relationship of the atrial myocardium, despite its negative inotropic effect, which is attributable to the solvent. It therefore differs fundamentally from the effects of flecainide on this important physiological compensatory mechanism.

4.6 Diastolic effects under amiodarone

In contrast to flecainide, neither amiodarone nor the solvent appear to mediate any effects on diastolic function in the atrial myocardium investigated here.

4.7 Clinical relevance of the results

Both flecainide and amiodarone are important drugs in the treatment of cardiac arrhythmias, especially in the most common cardiac arrhythmia, atrial fibrillation. However, the two drugs differ in their suitable patient population. Flecainide is reserved for people without structural heart disease and with good pump function, i.e. on average younger people. It is also suitable for a "pill in the pocket" approach[21]. Based on the results of the CAST study, flecainide is contraindicated in people for whom the above does not apply[22]. Amiodarone has proved its worth here, as it has hardly any cardiodepressive properties, but does have a number of extracardiac side effects. For this reason, amiodarone is more commonly used in people with pre-existing cardiac damage[(21) -48].

The results of this study confirm this approach. They are also consistent with the increased mortality under flecainide therapy described in the literature. For the first time, a deterioration of diastolic function in human atrial myocardium could also be demonstrated. For this reason, it seems sensible to monitor diastolic function regularly before and during flecainide therapy. The deterioration in CFB and the negative inotropic effect also suggest that this could lead to a symptomatic deterioration and further limitation of exercise tolerance even in patients with only mild cardiac insufficiency.

In contrast, amiodarone had no worsening effect on diastolic function and CFB in the experiments conducted as part of this study. The negative inotropic effects observed were primarily due to the solvent. The clinical applicability of amiodarone, especially in the acute setting, could be improved by using a different, less cardiodepressant solvent. Solutions based on cyclodextrin could be promising for this purpose[64].

The results of this study confirmed the use of amiodarone as a first-line antiarrhythmic agent in heart failure. Flecainide nevertheless has its place in people with good cardiac function, as it has a significantly more favourable side-effect profile than amiodarone.

CHAPTER 5

Tables

5.1 Flecainide CHP interventions

n = 13

Table 6:

Mean values	BL	10^{-8}M	10^{-7}M	10^{-6}M	$3*10^{-6}$M	10^{-5}M	10^{-4}M
Force [%]	100,00	94,03	87,60	82,48	71,55	49,37	21,16
SEM ±	0,00	1,98	2,74	3,31	5,39	8,09	4,85
Diast. [%]	100,00	98,79	99,65	95,14	89,84	89,37	99,47
SEM ±	0,00	2,94	5,39	5,85	6,96	8,02	16,72
RT50 [ms]	105,00	101,58	103,92	105,17	91,18	93,64	112,58
SEM ±	6,54	6,75	6,55	6,96	6,24	12,41	15,89
RT90 [ms]	188,33	180,00	185,00	195,00	200,00	201,67	200,00
SEM ±	7,26	10,00	18,03	18,93	15,28	24,55	26,46

5.2 Flecainide KWK - controls

n = 9

Table 7:

Mean values	BL	10^{-8}M	10^{-7}M	10^{-6}M	$3*10^{-6}$M	10^{-5}M	10^{-4}M
Force [%]	100,00	104,49	97,79	95,88	97,06	89,46	86,68
SEM ±	0,00	6,11	3,22	4,73	5,63	7,37	9,02
Diast. [%]	100,00	94,64	87,68	92,00	88,56	88,53	86,97
SEM ±	0,00	1,89	2,46	2,90	2,80	4,58	3,50
RT50 [ms]	84,86	95,29	93,25	102,25	94,14	94,14	98,00
SEM ±	4,87	11,12	8,89	9,62	9,83	12,43	13,24
RT90 [ms]	186,67	184,67	180,67	191,33	179,67	183,00	187,00
SEM ±	13,33	17,03	15,01	12,72	17,70	18,50	17,95

5.3 Amiodarone CHP interventions

n = 8

Table 8:

Mean values	BL	10^{-8}M	10^{-7}M	10^{-6}M	10^{-5}M	10^{-4}M	10^{-3}M
Force [%]	100,00	92,38	82,63	78,50	63,75	44,57	26,14
SEM ±	0,00	2,43	4,33	5,67	6,16	9,46	5,14
Diast. [%]	100,00	93,86	89,00	84,29	79,43	71,00	68,50
SEM ±	0,00	2,68	5,00	6,51	8,34	10,84	12,28
RT50 [ms]	82,44	82,67	83,46	84,59	85,85	90,11	81,91
SEM ±	4,42	5,50	4,25	6,59	11,47	14,29	6,89
RT90 [ms]	184,80	186,72	192,58	196,26	205,38	187,18	200,50
SEM ±	15,80	17,13	16,64	17,34	19,48	23,44	28,44

5.4 Amiodarone KWK - solvent

n = 6

Table 9:

Mean values	BL	10^{-8}M	10^{-7}M	10^{-6}M	10^{-5}M	10^{-4}M	10^{-3}M
Force [%]	100,00	101,00	102,00	103,50	90,83	60,83	18,50
SEM ±	0,00	2,48	3,42	8,67	6,85	9,26	8,55
Diast. [%]	100,00	89,83	80,33	74,83	81,40	80,80	76,60
SEM ±	0,00	4,50	7,86	11,18	3,67	5,81	6,02
RT50 [ms]	88,78	91,59	92,84	96,61	95,79	111,55	107,25
SEM ±	12,47	11,50	12,74	12,86	13,24	28,23	21,12
RT90 [ms]	169,85	177,80	179,25	180,68	178,57	180,26	214,50
SEM ±	19,92	19,83	19,98	18,22	18,30	22,83	35,50

5.5 Flecainide KFB - interventions

n = 7

Table 10:

Mean values	BL	1 Hz	1.5 Hz	2 Hz	2.5 Hz	3 Hz	1 Hz (end)
Force [%]	100,00	98,52	78,98	72,09	58,37	49,77	87,91
SEM ±	0,00	3,95	4,13	6,37	6,33	5,33	8,98
Diast. [%]	100,00	97,98	98,87	109,65	112,51	125,23	115,52
SEM ±	0,00	8,49	11,27	11,84	10,92	10,08	11,77
RT50 [ms]	72,64	72,42	70,92	69,50	58,33	56,57	74,21
SEM ±	7,09	8,30	6,94	6,23	6,18	5,00	7,25
RT90 [ms]	148,50	151,40	150,99	136,94	123,21	125,25	9,68
SEM ±	14,82	14,57	14,59	14,53	12,33	9,68	14,19

5.6 Flecainide KFB - controls

n = 6

Table 11:

Mean values	BL	1 Hz	1.5 Hz	2 Hz	2.5 Hz	3 Hz	1 Hz (end)
Force [%]	100,00	99,94	91,91	107,41	93,18	74,90	99,30
SEM ±	0,00	2,23	4,92	9,82	12,57	12,11	4,53
Diast. [%]	100,00	95,53	91,02	80,56	76,98	73,89	74,93
SEM ±	0,00	7,27	7,88	9,01	9,11	8,22	9,49
RT50 [ms]	59,60	60,17	58,82	57,17	51,61	52,04	66,24
SEM ±	7,37	7,29	7,37	6,32	5,98	6,29	8,59
RT90 [ms]	130,49	131,62	124,42	119,52	109,86	103,79	127,01
SEM ±	21,80	21,88	16,93	12,55	17,45	14,36	17,55

5.7 Amiodarone KFB - interventions

n = 6

Table 12:

Mean values	BL	1 Hz	1.5 Hz	2 Hz	2.5 Hz	3 Hz	1 Hz (end)
Force [%]	100,00	88,82	114,41	108,29	84,76	70,78	96,46

SEM ±	0,00	11,15	16,06	13,93	14,74	12,27	12,41
Diast. [%]	100,00	99,42	104,95	109,23	114,89	115,77	127,18
SEM ±	0,00	2,85	1,65	3,42	6,58	10,88	20,93
RT50 [ms]	57,71	61,22	72,61	73,03	71,28	60,22	73,88
SEM ±	4,28	4,24	10,33	8,16	5,63	3,24	11,54
RT90 [ms]	152,62	152,85	148,62	148,66	147,85	125,92	158,26
SEM ±	30,51	22,58	19,46	15,94	9,67	5,97	24,17

5.8 Amiodarone KFB - solvent

n = 5

Table 13:

Mean values	BL	1 Hz	1.5 Hz	2 Hz	2.5 Hz	3 Hz	1 Hz (end)
Force [%]	100,00	84,77	96,80	100,55	69,86	52,96	79,96
SEM ±	0,00	3,50	0,78	2,25	7,60	9,58	8,02
Diast. [%]	100,00	110,69	112,38	110,15	106,72	118,35	108,74
SEM ±	0,00	14,06	15,91	20,57	21,35	18,51	37,72
RT50 [ms]	63,15	57,77	70,52	69,92	72,01	60,95	76,71
SEM ±	10,69	6,86	12,27	11,91	9,60	10,92	8,52
RT90 [ms]	149,40	141,42	143,91	141,58	153,24	122,58	166,87
SEM ±	27,03	25,02	23,25	20,42	13,18	19,27	20,24

CHAPTER 6

Bibliography

1. Blanchard EM, Smith GL, Allen DG, Alpert NR. The effects of 2,3-butanedione monoxime on initial heat, tension, and aequorin light output of ferret papillary muscles. European Journal of Physiology 416(1-2), 219-221 (1990).

2. Mulieri LA, Hasenfuss G, Ittleman F, Blanchard EM, Alpert NR. Protection of human left ventricular myocardium from cutting injury with 2,3-butanedione monoxime. Circulation Research 65(5), 1441-1449 (1989).

3. Gwathmey JK, Hajjar RJ, Solaro RJ. Contractile deactivation and uncoupling of crossbridges. Effects of 2,3-butanedione monoxime on mammalian myocardium. Circulation Research 69(5), 1280-1292 (1991).

4. Phillips RM, Altschuld RA. 2,3-Butanedione 2-monoxime (BDM) induces calcium release from canine cardiac sarcoplasmic reticulum. Biochemical and Biophysical Research Communications 229(1), 154-157 (1996).

5. Solaro RJ. Mechanisms of the Frank-Starling law of the heart: the beat goes on. Biophysical Journal 93, 4095-4096 (2007).

6. Pagel C, Pieske B, Kirbel TH, Influence of the antiarrhythmic drugs flecainide and amiodarone on contractile function and the force-frequency relationship of the heart.
Göttingen (2009).

7. Latini R, Connoly SJ, Kates RE. Myocardial disposition of amiodarone in the dog. Journal of Pharmacology and Experimental Therapeutics 224, 603-608 (1983).

8. Hoth M., Wischmeyer E. Duale Reihe Physiologie: Elektrophysiologie des Herzens. 2nd edition. Stuttgart: Thieme, 74-83 (2012).

9. Nerbonne, JM, Kass RS. Molecular physiology of cardiac repolarisation. Physiological reviews 85, 1205-1253 (2005).

10. Fabiato A. Calcium-induced release of calcium from the cardiac sarcoplasmic reticulum. The American journal of physiology 245, C1-14 (1983).

11. Luis F. Santana, Edward P. Cheng, W. Jonathan Lederer, How does the shape of the cardiac action potential control calcium signalling and contraction in the heart? Journal of Molecular and Cellular Cardiology 49(6), 901-903 (2010).

12. Periasamy, M, Kalyanasundaram A. SERCA pump isoforms: their role in calcium transport and disease. Muscle & nerve 35, 430-442 (2007).

13. Kane C, Couch L, Terracciano CMN. Excitation-contraction coupling of human induced pluripotent

stem cell-derived cardiomyocytes. Frontiers in Cell and Developmental Biology 3, 59 (2015).

14. Pieske B, Maier LS, Bers DM, Hasenfuss G. Ca handling and sarcoplasmic reticulum Ca content in isolated failing and nonfailing human myocardium. Circulation Research 85, 38-45 (1999).

15. Bassani RA, Mattiazzi A, Bers DM: CaMK-II is responsible for activity-dependent acceleration of relaxation in rat ventricular myocytes. American Journal of Physiology 268, H 703-712 (1995).

16. Rettig J. Duale Reihe Physiologie: Grundlagen der Muskelphysiologie. 2nd edition. Stuttgart: Thieme, 57-64 (2012).

17. Gordon AM, Homsher E, Regnier M. Regulation of contraction in striated muscle. Physiological reviews 80, 853-924 (2000).

18. Andrikopoulos GK, Pastromas S, Tzeis S. Flecainide: Current status and perspectives in arrhythmia management. World Journal of Cardiology 7(2), 76-85 (2015).

19. Hwang HS, Hasdemir C, Laver D, Mehra D, Turhan K, Faggioni M, Yin H, Knollmann BC. Inhibition of cardiac Ca2+ release channels (RyR2) determines efficacy of that I antiarrhythmic drugs in catecholaminergic polymorphic ventricular tachycardia. Circulation: Arrhythmia and Electrophysiology 4(2), 128-35 (2011).

20. Bannister ML, Thomas NL, Sikkel MB, Mukherjee S, Maxwell C, MacLeod KT, George CH, Williams AJ. The mechanism of flecainide action in CPVT does not involve a direct effect on RyR2. Circulation Research 116(8), 1324-35 (2015).

21. Kirchhof P, Benussi S, Kotecha D, Ahlsson D, Atar D, Casadei B, Castella M, Diener HC et al. 2016 ESC Guidelines for the management of atrial fibrillation developed in collaboration with EACTS, European Heart Journal 37(38), 2893-2962 (2016).

22. Echt DS, Liebson PR, Mitchell LB, Peters RW, Obias-Manno D, Barker AH, Arensberg D, Baker A, Friedman L, Greene HL. Mortality and morbidity in patients receiving encainide, flecainide, or placebo. The Cardiac Arrhythmia Suppression Trial. New England Journal of Medicine 324(12), 781-788 (1991).

23. Aliot E, Capucci A, Crijns HJ, Goette A, Tamargo J. Twenty-five years in the making: flecainide is safe and effective for the management of atrial fibrillation. Europace 13(2), 161-173 (2011).

24. Martinez-Marcos FJ, Garcla-Garmendia JL, Ortega-Carpio A, Fernändez-Gömez JM, Santos JM, Camacho C. Comparison of intravenous flecainide, propafenone, and amiodarone for conversion of acute atrial fibrillation to sinus rhythm. The American Journal of Cardiology 86(9), 950-953 (2000).

25. Ekiz A, Kaya B, Bornaun H, Acar DK, Avci ME, Bestel A, Yildirim G. Flecainide as first-line treatment for foetal supraventriculartachycardia. Thejournal of maternal- fetal & neonatal medicine 31(4), 407-412 (2018).

26. Koch-Weser J, Blinks JR. The influence oft he interval between beats on myocardial contractility. Pharmacological Reviews 15(3), 601-652 (1963).

27. Münch G, Bölck B, Brixius K, Reuter H, Mehlhorn U, Bloch W, Schwinger RHG. SERCA2a activity

correlates with the force-frequency relationship in human myocardium. American Journal of Physiology. Heart and Circulatory Physiology 278(6), H1924-1932 (2000).

28. Piot C, LeMaire SA, Albat B, Seguin J, Nargeot J, Richard S. High frequency-induced upregulation of human cardiac calcium currents. Circulation 93(1), 120-8 (1996).

29. Sequeira V, van der Velden J. The Frank-Starling Law: a jigsaw of titin proportions. Biophysical Reviews 9(3), 259-267 (2017).

30. Schulze JJ, Knops J. Effects of flecainide on contractile force and electrophysiological parameters in cardiac muscle. Drug Research 32, 1025-1029 (1982).

31. Ito K, Nagafuchi K, Taga A, Yorikane R, Koike H. Possible involvement of altered Na+-Ca2+ exchange in negative inotropic effects of that I antiarrhythmic drugs on rabbit and rat ventricles. Journal of Cardiovascular Pharmacology 27, 355-361 (1996).

32. Watanabe H, Chopra N, Laver D, Hwang HS, Davies SS, Roach DE, Duff HJ, Roden DM, Wilde AAM, Knollmann BC. Flecainide prevents catecholaminergic polymorphic ventricular tachycardia in mice and humans. Nature Medicine 15(4), 380-383 (2009).

33. Hilliard FA, Steele DS, Laver D, Yang Z, Le Marchand SJ, Chopra N, Piston DW, Huke S, Knollmann BC. Flecainide inhibits arrhythmogenic Ca2+ waves by open state block of ryanodine receptor Ca2+ release channels and reduction of Ca2+ spark mass. Journal of Molecular Cellular Cardiology 48(2), 293 (2010).

34. Bannister ML, Alvarez-Laviada A, Thomas NL, Mason SA, Coleman S, du Plessis CL, Moran AT, Neill-Hall D, Osman H, Bagley MC, MacLeod KT, George CH, Williams AJ. Effect of flecainide derivatives on sarcoplasmic reticulum calcium release suggests a lack of direct action on the cardiac ryanodine receptor. British Journal of Pharmacology 173(15), 2446-2459 (2016).

35. Bannister ML, Thomas NL, Sikkel MB, Mukherjee S, Maxwell C, MacLeod KT, George CH, Williams AJ. The mechanism of flecainide action in CPVT does not involve a direct effect on RyR2. Circulation Research 10;116(8), 1324-35 (2015).

36. Curran J, Louch WE. Linking ryanodine receptor Ca2+ leak and Na+ current in heart: a day in the life of flecainide. Acta Physiologica (Oxf). 214(3), 300-302 (2015).

37. Kihara Y, Inoko M, Hatakeyama N, Momose Y, Sasayama S. Mechanisms of Negative Inotropic Effects of Class Ic Antiarrhythmic Agents: Comparative Study of the Effects of Flecainide and Pilsicainide on Intracellular Calcium Handling in Dog Ventricular Myocardium. Journal of Cardiovascular Pharmacology 27(1), 42-51 (1996).

38. Scamps F, Undrovinas A, Vassort G. Inhibition of ICa in single frag cardiac cells by quinidine, flecainide, ethmozin, and ethacizin. American Journal of Physiology 256(3), C549-559 (1993).

39. Homma M, Kuga K, Doki K, Katori K, Yamaguchi I, Sugibayashi K, Kohda Y. Assessment of serum flecainide trough levels in patients with tachyarrhythmia. Journal of Pharmacy and Pharmacology 57(1), 47-51 (2005).

40. Kowey PR. Pharmacological Effects of Antiarrhythmic Drugs: Review and Update. JAMA Internal

Medicine 158(4), 325-332 (1998).

41. Melgari D, Zhang Y, El Harchi A, Dempsey CE, Hancox JC. Molecular basis of hERG potassium channel blockade by the class Ic antiarrhythmic flecainide. Journal of Molecular and Cellular Cardiology 86, 42-53 (2015).

42. Yue L, Feng JL, Wang Z, Nattel S. Effects of ambasilide, quinidine, flecainide and verapamil on ultra-rapid delayed rectifier potassium currents in canine atrial myocytes. Cardiovascular Research 46(1), 151-161 (2000).

43. Yamashita T, Nakajima T, Hamada E, Hazama H, Omata M, Kurachi Y. Flecainide inhibits the transient outward current in atrial myocytes isolated from the rabbit heart. Journal of Pharmacology and Experimental Therapeutics 274(1), 315-321 (1995).

44. Wang Z, Fermini B, Nattel S. Effects of flecainide, quinidine, and 4-aminopyridine on transient outward and ultrarapid delayed rectifier currents in human atrial myocytes. Journal of Pharmacology and Experimental Therapeutics 272(1), 184-196 (1995).

45. Olsson SB, Edvardsson N. Clinical electrophysiologic study of antiarrhythmic properties of flecainide: acute intraventricular delayed conduction and prolonged repolarisation in regularly paced and premature beats using intracardiac monophasic action potentials with programmed stimulation. American Heart Journal 102: 864- 871 (1981).

46. Schwinger RH, Böhm M, Koch A, Uhlmann R, Überfuhr P, Kreuzer E, Reichart B, Erdmann E. Force-frequency-relation in human atrial and ventricular myocardium. Molecular and Cellular Biochemistry 17;119(1-2), 73-78 (1993).

47. Wang GK, Russell C, Wang S. State-dependent Block of Wild-type and Inactivation- deficient Na+ Channels by Flecainide. The Journal of General Physiology 122(3), 365-374 (2003).

48. Elsa-Grace Giardina, Passman R. Amiodarone: Clinical uses. Uptodate (2018). Post TW, ed. UpToDate. Waltham, MA: UpToDate Inc. http://www.uptodate.com (Accessed 20 Aug 2018).

49. Goldschlager N, Epstein AE, Naccarelli GV, Olshansky B, Singh B, Collard HR, Murphy E. A Practical Guide for Clinicians Who Treat Patients with Amiodarone: 2007 Heart Rhythm 4(12), 1590 (2007).

50. Al-Khatib SM, Stevenson WG, Ackerman MJ, Gillis AM, Bryant WJ, Hlatky MA, Callans DJ, Granger CB, Curtis AB, Hammill SC, Deal BJ, Joglar JA, Dickfeld T, Kay GN, Field ME, Matlock DD, Fonarow GC, Myerburg RJ, Page RL. 2017 AHA/ACC/HRS Guideline for Management of Patients With Ventricular Arrhythmias and the Prevention of Sudden Cardiac Death: A Report of the American College of Cardiology/American Heart Association Task Force on Clinical Practice Guidelines and the Heart Rhythm Society. Circulation 2017, https://doi.Org/10.1161/CIR.0000000000000550 (Accessed 15 July 2018).

51. Priori SG, Blomström-Lundqvist C, Mazzanti A, Blom N, Borggrefe M, Camm J, Elliott PM, Fitzsimons D, Hatala R, Hindricks G, Kirchhof P, Kjeldsen K, Kuck KH, Hernandez-Madrid A, Nikolaou N, Norekväl TM, Spaulding C, Van Veldhuisen DJ. 2015 ESC Guidelines for the management of patients with ventricular arrhythmias and the prevention of sudden cardiac death: The Task Force for the Management of Patients with Ventricular Arrhythmias and the Prevention of Sudden Cardiac Death of the European Society of Cardiology (ESC). Endorsed by: Association for European Paediatric and

Congenital Cardiology (AEPC). European Heart Journal 36(41), 2793-2867 (2015).

52. Massie BM, Fisher SG, Radford M, Deedwania PC, Singh BN, Fletcher RD, Singh SN. Effect of amiodarone on clinical status and left ventricular function in patients with congestive heart failure. CHF-STAT Investigators. Circulation 15;94(10), 2668 (1996). "

53. van Tellingen O, Beijnen JH, Verweij J, Scherrenburg EJ, Nooijen WJ, Sparreboom A. Rapid Esterase-sensitive Breakdown of Polysorbate 80 and Its Impact on the Plasma Pharmacokinetics of Docetaxel and Metabolites in Mice. Clinical Cancer Research 5(10), 2918-2924 (1999).

54. Pfisterer M, Burkart F, Müller-Brand J, Kiowski W. Important differences between short- and long-term hemodynamic effects of amiodarone in patients with chronic ischemic heart disease at rest and during ischemia-induced left ventricular dysfunction. Journal of the American College of Cardiology 5(5), 1205-1211 (1985).

55. Suzuki T, Morishima M, Kato S, Ueda N, Honjo H, Kamiya K. Atrial selectivity in Na+channel blockade by acute amiodarone. Cardiovascular Research 98(1), 136- 144 (2013).

56. Mason JW, Hondeghem LM, Katzung BG. Block of inactivated sodium channels and of depolaisation-induced automaticity in guinea pig papillary muscle by amiodarone. Circulation Research 55, 277-285 (1984).

57. Nattel S, Talajic M, Quantz M, De Roode M. Frequency-dependent effects of amiodarone on atrio-ventricular nodal function and slow-channel action potentials: Evidence for calcium channel blocking activity. Circulation 76, 442-449 (1987).

58. Lubic SP, Nguyen KPV, Dave B, Giacomini JC. Antiarrhythmic agent amiodarone posesses calcium channel blocker properties. Journal of Cardiovasc Phamnacology 24, 707-714(1994).

59. Drvota V, Häggblad J, Blange I, Magnusson Y, Sylven S. The effect of amiodarone on the beta-adrenergic receptor is due to a downregulation of receptor protein and not to a receptor-ligand interaction. Biochemical and Biophysical Research Communications 255(2), 515-520 (1999).

60. Vassy R, Starzec A, Yin Y, Nicolas P, Perret GY. Amiodarone has exclusively non-genomic action on cardiac beta-adrenoceptor regulation. European Journal of Pharmacology 408(3), 227-232 (2000).

61. Munoz A, Karila P, Gallay P, Zettelmeier F, Messner P, Mery M, Grolleau R. A randomised hemodynamic comparison of intravenous amiodarone with and without Tween 80. European Heart Journal 9(2), 142-148 (1988).

62. Platou ES, Refsum H. Acute electrophysiologic and blood pressure effects of amiodarone and its solvent in the dog. Acta Pharmacol Toxicol (Copenh). 58(3), 163-168 (1986).

63. Somberg JC, Cao W, Cvetanovic I, Ranade V, Molnar J. Pharmacology and toxicology of a new aqueous formulation of intravenous amiodarone (Amio- Aqueous) compared with Cordarone IV. American Journal of Therapeutics 12(1), 9- 16(2005).

64. Lindquist DE, Rowe AS, Heidel E, Fleming T, Yates JR. Evaluation of the Hemodynamic Effects of Intravenous Amiodarone Formulations During the Maintenance Phase Infusion. Annals of Pharmacotherapy 49(12), 1317-1321 (2015).

65. Yasaka WJ, Eichbaum FW, Oga S. Antiarrhythmic effects of solvents: III Effects of propylene glycol and benzyl alcohol on contractile force of isolated rabbit heart. Cardiovascular Research 13(12), 717-722 (1979).

66. Hoth M., Wischmeyer E. Duale Reihe Physiologie: Steuerung der Herzätigkeit. 2nd edition. Stuttgart: Thieme, 100-104 (2012).

67. Rosen MR, Bigger JT, Breithardt G, Brown AM, Camm AJ, Carmeliet E, Fozzard HA, Hoffman BF, Janse MJ, Lazzara R, et al. The Sicilian gambit. A new approach to the Classification of antiarrhythmic drugs based on their actions on arrhythmogenic mechanisms. Task Force of the Working Group on Arrhythmias of the European Society of Cardiology. Circulation. 84(4), 1831-1851 (1991).

68. Burashnikov A, Di Diego JM, Sicouri S, Ferreira M, Carlsson L, Antzelevitch C. Atrial-Selective Effects of Chronic Amiodarone in the Management of Atrial Fibrillation. Heart Rhythm. 5(12), 1735-1742 (2008).

69. Bisping E, Pagel C, Wilken A, Toischer K, Pieske B. The antiarrhythmic agent flecainide induced diastolic dysfunction, but not amiodarone. Wiener klinische Wochenschrift 120(15-16), A52-A52. (2008).

70. Watanabe Y, Kimura J. Inhibitory effect of amiodarone on Na+/Ca2+ exchange current in guinea-pig cardiac myocytes. British Journal of Pharmacology 131(1), 80- 84 (2000).

71. Watanabe Y, Matsuoka I, Kimura J. Chronic Administration of Amiodarone Does Not Affect Na+/Ca2+ Exchange Current in Guinea Pig Cardiac Ventricular Myocytes. The Japanese Journal of Pharmacology 90, 21-27 (2002).

72. Koss KL, Kranias EG. Phospholamban: a prominent regulator of myocardial contractility. Circulation Research 79, 1059-1063 (1996).

73. Bai Y, Jones PP, Guo J, Zhong X, Clark RB, Zhou Q, Wang R, Vallmitjana A, Benitez R, Hove-Madsen L, Semeniuk L, Guo A, Song LS, Duff HJ, Chen SRW. Phospholamban Knockout Breaks Arrhythmogenic Ca2+ Waves and Suppresses Catecholaminergic Polymorphic Ventricular Tachycardia in Mice. Circulation Research 113(5), 10(2013).

FSC
www.fsc.org
MIX
Papier | Fördert gute Waldnutzung
FSC® C083411

Kolibri 360 GmbH
Ferdinand-Jühlke-Straße 7
99095 Erfurt, Deutschland
produktsicherheit@kolibri360.de

Druck:
CPI Druckdienstleistungen GmbH
im Auftrag der
Kolibri 360 GmbH
Ferdinand-Jühlke-Str. 7
99095 Erfurt